DHARMA PARENTING

DHARMA
PARENTING

Understand Your Child's
Brilliant Brain for Greater Happiness,
Health, Success, and Fulfillment

Robert Keith Wallace, PhD
Frederick Travis, PhD

A TarcherPerigee Book

tarcherperigee

An imprint of Penguin Random House LLC
375 Hudson Street
New York, New York 10014

Most TarcherPerigee books are available at special quantity discounts for bulk
purchase for sales promotions, premiums, fund-raising, and educational needs.
Special books or book excerpts also can be created to fit specific needs. For details,
write: SpecialMarkets@penguinrandomhouse.com.

ISBN 9780399185007

Printed in the United States of America
10 9 8 7 6 5 4 3 2 1

Book design by Pauline Neuwirth

To our Dear Families
with Love and Appreciation

CONTENTS

APPENDICES 255

ACKNOWLEDGMENTS

IT'S OUR JOY to thank our wives, Samantha and Nita, for helping to shape the structure of the book, editing many drafts of the manuscript, and adding the fruit of their experience in the Notes from Mom. We especially want to acknowledge and thank our editor, Mitch Horowitz, for recognizing the value of Dharma Parenting, and for his guidance at every step.

Special thanks goes to Bob Roth for his wise suggestions and help, and to Ted and Danielle Wallace for hosting the first class on Dharma Parenting, and for their always helpful suggestions. We also thank Cindy Buck for editing earlier versions of the book, Andrew Sternberg for his knowledgeable description of the self-pulse technique, and Annalisa Miller for her wonderfully applicable Winnie-the-Pooh analogy of body types. Finally, we thank the Enlightened Bestseller group of Chris and Janet Attwood, Marci Shimoff, and Geoff Affleck for their expertise and generous encouragement.

DHARMA
PARENTING

INTRODUCTION TO DHARMA PARENTING

DHARMA PARENTING IS A UNIQUE approach to raising happy and successful children. It starts with the understanding that kids are people with their own strengths and weakness, their own gifts and preferences. Dharma Parenting provides you with simple tools to help your children discover *who they are and what they can become.*

Dharma is a concept found in Eastern traditions. The word "dharma" comes from the Sanskrit verb *dhri*, which means to "uphold" or "support." Our dharma is our path in life—the lifestyle that supports our personal growth, happiness, success, and fulfillment. Dharma is different at different ages, and for different children. One child learns quickly and forgets quickly, while another learns slowly and forgets slowly. One may be content to work alone for long periods of time; another wants to be surrounded by friends. If we are lucky, we find our dharma early in life.

For example, we know a brilliant second-year college student who wants to teach high school math. He feels that he was born to be a teacher—his parents were both teachers, and he has been tutoring classmates since third grade. He tells us there's nothing as satisfying as his friends' "Aha!" when they finally "get" what he's trying to teach them. It's clear that teaching is his dharma. Two of his college professors, however, were shocked when he revealed his career goal. One responded by telling him to get a PhD: "You could do brilliant theoretical work!" And his computer science teacher said, "You could become a world-class programmer and be a millionaire before you're twenty-five!" Both of these professors were projecting their own talents and desires onto the student, instead of encouraging his special aptitudes and interest. Rather than help him find his own path, they wanted him to travel down theirs. The tools of Dharma Parenting allow us to recognize and nurture our children's unique path in life: what they're good at, what they enjoy, what helps them grow. In addition, these tools help us understand each of the stages of brain development, from birth to adulthood, so our parenting takes into account our children's developmental level—not demanding things that they cannot yet accomplish, but always gently encouraging them to use more of their potential.

Dharma Parenting tools help us find our own dharma as a parent. Did you ever wish that babies came with manuals? It's so much easier to use a new gadget when there's an instruction manual! Parenting is tremendously complex and often hopelessly confusing. Understanding the principles of brain/body types and the stages of brain development will empower you to apply Dharma Parenting tools in a variety of changing situations. In other words, you will be able to begin to fulfill your dharma as a parent.

Dharma Parenting incorporates six parenting tools that apply to children of all age groups. They're easy to remember using the word "dharma" as an acronym:

> **D**iscover your child's, and your own, brain/body type
> **H**eal yourself
> **A**ttention and **a**ppreciation
> **R**outines to improve family dynamics
> **M**anage **m**eltdowns and cultivate better behavior
> **A**nticipate and **a**dapt

Let's see how these tools might be applied in a specific situation.

> *Six-year-old Ryan storms into the kitchen, his blue eyes welling with tears, cheeks flaming red, as he flings his game box onto the floor, cracking its screen.*
> *"This game is stupid. I hate it!" the boy screams, and runs out of the room, leaving his mother shaken. What can I do? she wonders. How do I handle his rage?*

Ryan is a bright, energetic child who can be perfectly agreeable and normal for days, until some small thing throws him into a violent tantrum. Lately, both of Ryan's parents have noticed his growing tendency to overreact, almost to *overheat*—mentally, physically, and emotionally—and they are increasingly concerned. What's causing this alarming behavior? What is the cure? Is it time to find a child psychologist? Is it just a case of "boys will be boys"? Does he need medication?

THE FIRST TOOL—D: DISCOVER YOUR CHILD'S, AND YOUR OWN, BRAIN/BODY TYPE

Your brain/body type includes (1) your inherited tendencies and preferences that have been hardwired from birth, also known as our "body type," (2) the state of balance or imbalance of your body type, and (3) your changing brain connections, which are constantly being shaped by ongoing experiences as well the stage of your brain development. Ryan appears to be a particular brain/body type that is susceptible to anger. Also, Ryan is six years old. His brain is wired to be a sensory-motor machine that sees the world very concretely. If a video machine doesn't work, it should be thrown out. So when his game box stopped working, he became upset and threw it away because of the *state* of his brain/body type as well as his age-related brain connections.

One brain/body type responds with impatience and anger. Another might respond with nervousness and fear. A third type might not respond at all. The combination of inherent tendencies and personal brain development determines how everyone responds.

In chapter 1 you will learn about the basic characteristics of each type and you can take a short quiz to help you figure out your child's brain/body type, as well as your own and the rest of your family's. In chapter 2, we will discuss interactions between family members with different brain/body types. In the last section of this chapter, we'll explore in greater detail how the brain changes during the first two decades of life and how these changes shape behavior.

THE SECOND TOOL—H: HEAL YOURSELF

If you are tired or stressed, you might well respond very much like Ryan's mother did. She started to yell—after all, it was an expensive video game. But once you and your child begin to yell, the situation explodes into chaos and nothing gets resolved.

We understand that you're a parent 24-7, and with all the demands of raising kids, there may not seem to be time for healing yourself. But you've got to remain aware of your own needs—for your children's sake as well as your own.

THE THIRD TOOL—A: ATTENTION AND APPRECIATION

If Ryan's mom or dad had sat down with him and helped him better understand how to play the game, and if they had congratulated him on how well he was doing *before* he became so frustrated, his blowup might have been avoided. Childhood is a roller-coaster ride of growth and development, propelled by massive transformations in the child's brain connections. Parental attention during these years is critical for your child to learn how to work in groups and develop self-esteem, social skills, a sense of right and wrong, respect for others, and even critical and creative thinking.

Your attention is immensely important. Children are not static objects; they are constantly growing in response to each new experience. By appreciating each new accomplishment, you are supporting their developing sense of self and ability to interact with the world.

THE FOURTH TOOL—R: ROUTINES TO IMPROVE FAMILY DYNAMICS

Established routines—bedtime routines, dining room routines, or shopping routines—give children a sense of security. They know what is expected of them in each situation. Routines break up a long day into meaningful chunks and give your child a feeling of being in control.

Another valuable routine is family meetings—a designated time to talk about issues in a calm and supportive setting. This would be an ideal setting for Ryan's parents to help him figure out what to do when his toys don't work: for example, put them on a special shelf, tell Mom or Dad what's wrong with them, and then play Mr. Fix-It together.

THE FIFTH TOOL—M: MANAGE MELTDOWNS AND CULTIVATE BETTER BEHAVIOR

This tool consists of six recommendations, all starting with the letter C.

1. **Check in** with yourself and with your child
2. **Comfort** your child
3. **Change** brain states
4. **Choices**
5. **Consequences**
6. **Coach**

Let's apply these six C's to Ryan's situation:

Check in with yourself and with your child. Ryan's parents first need to determine their own brain states. For example: Are their emotions on edge? Did they skip lunch and are now famished and irritated?

Next, they need to check in with their son. Was the video game too difficult for him? Was he overheated or hungry or both? Is he having problems at school? Is he sleeping badly? Ryan is six years old; this means that the prefrontal "executive" circuits of his brain have not developed yet. At this age, he can't even begin to comprehend such adult abstractions as "Do you know how much that game costs?"

Comfort your child. Your child knows that something is wrong. The thinking centers of his brain are overwhelmed with strong emotions. A long, warm hug or just a touch on the shoulder reassures him that everything is going to be okay. Comforting your child is the basis for your success in following the C's. It lets him know that some part of his world is loving and supportive, no matter how badly he's feeling.

Change the brain state. The first thing Ryan needs is to cool down his overheated brain. When your child overreacts, it is because the primitive emotional brain has taken over. Reason is simply not available at that moment. Strong passionate emotions dominate, and the child can only respond impulsively. Ryan needs help so he can switch from being dominated by his irrational, emotional brain to being able to use his reflective, thinking brain. Even moving to another part of the house can help him begin to settle down. We will talk more about meltdowns and temper tantrums in chapter 6.

Choices. Once Ryan is calm, his mom and dad can offer him concrete choices—for example, "The next time your game doesn't work, bring it to one of us so we can fix it." By helping Ryan reflect on his actions, his parents are showing him how to deal with frustration in the future and allowing him to exercise his executive brain circuits so they will be more available.

Consequences. Ryan needs to be held accountable for his actions. His tantrum had a natural consequence: he broke his game box, so he can no longer play with it. At the family meeting, Ryan and his parents can now discuss how he can earn a new one.

Coach. As a parent, you are your child's life coach. What do coaches do? In sports, they ensure that their athletes *train before the game* so they will be successful in competition. The coach watches the play and will take players out of the game if they're becoming overheated or emotional. Coaches teach fair play and good values. They sum up each experience so the players gain positive insight into future situations.

As coaches, we model correct behavior. Neurons in the brain called "mirror neurons" help children model what they see. Show your child how you might deal with the situation. If he makes a mistake, help him figure out how to fix it and how to avoid it next time.

THE SIXTH TOOL—A: ANTICIPATE AND ADAPT

Whether you're focused on nurturing your child's talents or working to ensure that family life moves smoothly through the day, part of your dharma as a parent is to anticipate your family's needs. Once you are familiar with the first five Dharma Parenting tools, you will naturally find yourself looking ahead to see how you can use those tools to avoid crises. Even so, despite your best efforts, unexpected situations will come up. You will need to adapt to the situation, using your best judgment.

DHARMA PARENTING TOOLS ARE DIFFERENT WHEN APPLIED TO DIFFERENT AGE GROUPS

Throughout the first twenty-five years of life, your child's brain is a work in progress. With each change in brain structure and function, he begins to see the world more globally, gets better at controlling impulses, begins to see consequences, and grows in understanding abstract ideas. Dharma Parenting tools, therefore, have different characters in the four major stages of brain development. We systematically discuss the relationship between brain development and Dharma Parenting tools in the last four chapters.

FROM BIRTH TO THREE YEARS

Children are born with their brain unassembled. At birth, the infant does not see you or hear your soothing words—your baby sees and hears only disconnected bursts of light and sound. Within the first three years, brain connections grow exponentially and children grow in the ability to interact with the world. By six months of age, the visual system develops and the child sees objects in the world around them. By two years, the hearing system develops and the child connects individual sounds into the flow of speech. During this time, Dharma Parenting tools support the developing brain and help your child begin to interact with the world.

FROM FOUR TO NINE YEARS

Four to nine are the school years. During this time, your child has the highest number of connections between brain cells

that he will ever have. Also, the left and right hemispheres of
the brain are being connected. This is the time when the child
learns how to work in groups, how to take turns, and how to
follow rules. It's also the time of creative play—the child's
imagination transforms any object into many possibilities. At
this age, Dharma Parenting tools support the child's increasing ability to think and reflect on the world. Now you can
include the child when structuring guidelines and discussing
rules of family life.

FROM TEN TO SEVENTEEN YEARS

During the preteen and teenage years, 2 percent of all brain-
cell connections drop off each year in a natural "pruning" that
follows a "use it or lose it" rule. So many changes are happening so quickly that the brain your teenager wakes up with in
the morning is not the same brain he went to sleep with the
night before. The teen years are also a time when fatty layers
begin to be added to the prefrontal executive circuits. This
results in a speeding up of the flow of information in brain
areas responsible for long-term planning and ethical decision
making. The teenager is now beginning to think more abstractly. Rules are no longer absolute but have different meaning in different contexts. At this age, Dharma Parenting tools
help your teen make the transition from being a child to a
young adult.

FROM EIGHTEEN TO TWENTY-FIVE YEARS

Eighteen to twenty-five are the young adult years. The final
stroke of brain development occurs as neural pruning levels
off and connections with prefrontal executive brain circuits

fully mature. The result is that the young adult begins to think more broadly and more abstractly. Young adults can imagine alternative situations and consider each one separately and in detail. At this age, Dharma Parenting tools support your young adult stepping out on his own—using these tools to guide their own lives and eventually their own families.

WITH ALL THAT YOU HAVE TO DO, HOW CAN YOU POSSIBLY FIT THESE TOOLS INTO YOUR LIFE?

We understand that you have constant demands on your attention: work, meals, laundry, car pool, various lessons for your kids, and hundreds of other things. Your mind needs to go in many directions, at ninety miles an hour, every minute of the day. How can you possibly manage to remember all the Dharma Parenting tools and use them? Especially when your child is throwing a tantrum or grabbing the car keys and racing off to heave them down the toilet? It's just more pressure, trying to be a better parent—along with being a useful employee, a nutritionist, an on-time chauffeur, and a caring spouse.

Fred's oldest daughter is an avid cook, and recently she took a course on the most efficient use of a knife. She learned the best techniques to chop everything from asparagus to zucchini—but the first thing she learned was how to sharpen a knife.

This is a lesson for all of us: no matter what techniques we use, they won't do much good if our knife is dull. Techniques like Dharma Parenting improve our lives. But before we can put them into practice, we need to expand our basic ability to think and act. We can read all the books we want, but if we're stressed and overwhelmed, we won't be able to implement any of the great ideas we read about.

For the writers of this book, the ultimate parenting tool has been Transcendental Meditation (TM). We have both been meditating since college, and we've learned that the TM technique is a great preparation for life, and especially for the most demanding job of all—parenting. First of all, TM gives you twenty minutes of effortless and profound rest and rejuvenation twice a day. It allows your mind to completely settle down, so your accumulated knots of stress and tension can loosen and dissolve. It's an amazing way to start your morning—fresh, clear, and energized. And at the end of a stressful, demanding day, your afternoon meditation gives you the calm renewal you need before the demands of family time in the evening.

TM actually helps your brain function more coherently. After each meditation, your mind feels clearer; you see the big picture while simultaneously being able to focus on details. With regular twice-a-day practice, you start noticing that inner orderliness and energy are present more of the day, and become even stronger over time.

These three benefits—clearer thinking, relief from stress, and more energy—are invaluable for any parent. When you're more energetic at the same time that you're feeling calm and thinking clearly, you'll have the mental resources to implement the parenting tools in this book. And your job as a parent will be much easier if your children have the benefit of doing TM too. There's a children's technique that can be learned as early as age four, and your child can learn the adult sitting technique at ten. Kids need a good stress buster as much as we do, and their developing brains thrive on the greater orderliness and acuity that TM brings.

The ultimate gift that anyone can give their children is self-knowledge and self-awareness, which allows them to build their own happiness and success. This doesn't happen overnight, and requires both time and attention. As parents, we are not the architects of our children's brain. We do, however, influence brain development through the environment we create for our kids, and the mental challenges and emotional support we provide for them.

Please note: Throughout the book we use the term "brain/body type" and we would like both parents and children to understand that no one is limited by his or her brain/body type. The word "type" has become increasingly common in both the popular and scientific literature. For our purposes, we interpret it to mean "tendencies" rather than fixed characteristics.

DHARMA
PARENTING
TOOLS

CHAPTER 1

THE FIRST TOOL OF DHARMA PARENTING:
Discover Your Child's Brain/Body Type

KNOWLEDGE IS POWER. AND LEARNING your child's brain/ body type is the first step in developing positive parenting power by improving your parenting skills. Every child is a unique combination of individual tendencies. Sometimes parents understand and relate better to one offspring because that particular child shares similar inclinations and behavioral traits with them, while another child may seem a complete mystery. Scientists, therapists, and sociologists have studied individual differences and tendencies in an effort to understand these differences, and research has identified a variety of different types:

- Physical body types (ectomorph, mesomorph, and endomorph)
- Mental types (multiple intelligences)
- Emotional types (high/low emotional reactivity)
- Social types (high/low need for attachment)

- Behavioral types (high/low stress reactivity, types A and B)

Modern science has not yet, however, integrated this information into one holistic system of "typing" that can be used by health professionals, educators, and parents to *understand individual differences*. Ayurveda is an ancient system of natural medicine, which includes mind/body types as defined by distinct behavioral, biochemical, and physiological characteristics.

Dharma Parenting draws on the time-tested knowledge of Ayurveda's mind/body types and combines it with the latest understanding of how the brain is shaped by natural maturation and experience. These two factors—natural patterns of response and ongoing brain changes—contribute to what we call *brain/body types*, which are enormously useful for understanding your child's behavior.

Many of you have heard of Ayurveda from popular TV shows, health articles, or books. Originating in India, Ayurveda is the most ancient system of natural medicine. It includes a rich knowledge of the therapeutic use of plants, food, and spices, which modern science is now recognizing and researching in order to better deal with heart disease and cancer, among other disorders. Ayurveda defines physical, mental, emotional, social, and behavioral tendencies in terms of three main patterns, or brain/body types, which are traditionally called Vata (vah'tah), Pitta (pit'ah), and Kapha (kah'fah). (Appendix 1 gives fuller details on Maharishi Ayurveda.)

- The Vata body type is sensitive, always changing, and creative.
- The Pitta body type is dynamic, strong willed, and inquisitive.
- The Kapha body type is calm, steady, and kind.

NOTE FROM MOM

AROMATHERAPY: Aroma oils have become part of our mainstream culture—even dish soap, with its man-made fragrance, claims to revive our senses and calm our nerves. Be careful to use authentic aromatherapy oils, compounded according to traditional Ayurvedic specifications and not just dreamed up to satisfy the current trend. Maharishi Ayurveda aromatherapy has carefully investigated how aromas balance and improve our well-being and has created Calming Vata, Cooling Pitta, and Stimulating Kapha Aroma Oils using organic essential oils to keep everyone's brain/body type in good balance. Other favorites, which are great for kids older than six months and for grown-ups, are:

Slumber Time: Use this soothing aroma oil a half hour before bedtime to help settle your child (or yourself) into sleep.

Blissful Heart: This aroma oil is surely a preschool mom's best friend. We all know what it's like when a playdate is about to end—nobody wants to go home, and everyone is on the verge of tears! Avoid the agony and increase the bliss by using this aroma half an hour before it's time to leave.

Sniffle Free: The penetrating woodsy scent of this aroma oil will help to clear a stuffy nose, whether it's from a cold or allergies.

At any time of the day, your child's brain/body type can be either balanced or imbalanced, resulting in corresponding behavioral, emotional, and physical states. Understanding what triggers imbalance in your child will help you understand what they're experiencing and how to help them with their reactions. In addition, transformation in brain circuits occurring during childhood colors the way your child's natural tendencies are expressed. By attending to your child's brain/body type—his natural tendencies and changing brain connections—you'll be able to better understand what your child needs to be happy and successful.

THE TRADITIONAL AYURVEDA BODY TYPES

VATA BODY TYPE

Vata represents *movement*—our breath moving in and out of the lungs; our hands gesturing, stroking, gripping; our feet walking, running, dancing; our eyes opening, closing, and blinking; and our mouth laughing, speaking, and eating—with the many variations of each action. Vata children think fast, and their moods and energy levels change fast. Vata is compared to the wind: light and moving, cool and dry.

Physically, Vata types tend to be tall and on the thin side when young, or they can be small and delicate—you can almost see the wind blowing through them. Vata is cold, so they frequently suffer from cold hands or feet and must generally take extra care to keep warm. Vata is also dry, so Vata skin can be very dry or rough. They are energetic and move fast, but these kids are sprinters rather than long-distance runners, with bursts of energy rather than stamina. Their lithe bodies and artistic natures give them an edge in dance or gymnastics.

Vatas may have digestive problems. Have you ever tried to cook breakfast over a campfire in a strong wind? The fire is hot but not so steady—you can fry an egg quickly or toast a marshmallow, but you can't cook a pot of oatmeal or a stew. Vatas' digestion is irregular too: sometimes they're hungry, sometimes they're not. And they appreciate and tend to do better with a variety of small, light meals. A heavy meal of lasagna and bread, with strawberry shortcake and whipped cream for dessert, may clog up their system so they end up with a cold. Because Vata is dry, they can be prone to constipation, especially when traveling. Keeping your Vata child well hydrated and away from cold, dry foods will help.

Vatas are especially vulnerable in cold, windy weather. Winter hats are a must—something warm and snuggly and fun to wear. A Vata child catches cold easily in the winter, with lots of sneezing, a runny nose, and a dry cough. When your little Vata comes in from winter play, a warm drink and hot food will help them equilibrate. Hot soup and a warm sandwich will be a much better snack for them than crispy cookies or cold juice.

Traveling can be especially hard on Vata children, since by definition it involves lots of movement as well as lots of stimulation. Make sure they have familiar toys and blankets so they feel secure, and snacks and drinks so their restless Vata bodies are warmly nourished, and be sure to follow their usual daily routine before and after the trip.

The Vata mind is always moving. Most Vatas have extremely active minds and are blessed with great imagination and creativity. They are also quick to learn—but unfortunately, they are also quick to forget. They are particularly good at learning verbal skills, and as babies will generally speak quite early. It's their nature to enjoy talking and they do a lot of it, from babbling as babies to talking and texting as teens. They tend to overdo the multitasking and are easily distracted. Make sure that your Vata teen is absolutely convinced that cell phones and driving don't mix.

Vatas are *highly sensitive* to all sensory stimuli and must be protected from overstimulation. At the same time, this sensitivity makes it ideal for them to participate and excel in the arts. Encourage this gift with creative play ideas. When they are young, crayons and scissors, colored paper, feathers, pretty stones, and glue suit them much better than electronic games. Vatas tend to be very emotionally sensitive as well, and it's worth noting that one characteristic of Vata, which is frequently referred to in Ayurveda, is *euphoric*. When your Vata child is in good balance he will probably love to paint and dance, and will respond to songs and poetry. When they're out of balance, Vatas can be "high strung," nervous, or even fearful. High-energy or violent movies or video games may stimulate them almost out of control. Avoid them if you can, but if you can't, then be sure to turn everything off some hours before bedtime if you expect your Vata to be able to sleep.

Emotionally, the Vata child is enthusiastic and flexible and loves change. They are stimulating to be with because they are always discovering something new. Their attention is constantly moving from one topic to another, so it's good to gently help them focus. Always try to interest and charm, rather than force, your Vata child.

Even as teens and adults, Vatas tend to have *rapidly varying energy levels*, with bursts of energy, being very active and happy for quite some time, and then suddenly feeling exhausted or imbalanced. When they are little, monitor them carefully and make sure they take a break before they crash. As they grow up, helping them understand the qualities of their Vata brain/body type will enable them to learn to start monitoring themselves.

Vatas can be scattered and indecisive, so the stability of a good *daily routine* is vital to help them stay in balance. A well-thought-out routine helps keep them in balance and at their peak. This means specific routines for sleep, play, exercise, schoolwork, and meals. Since *rest is one of the most critical variables* for a Vata, it's important to establish a solid routine at bedtime. Begin early with a warm, soothing bath, use Vata pacifying aroma oils, read an uplifting and calming story, and play soft music. Do everything you can to create a quiet and enticing environment before you even try to get your Vata child to sleep.

It's best not to give Vatas too many choices. They love variety but can have a hard time making decisions or may decide too quickly on impulse or whim. And when they do decide on something, they often change their minds minutes later. Make life easier for everyone and don't offer too many *or* too few choices. Always remember that your sensitive Vata child will naturally have definite likes and dislikes. Try to go with the flow of their discerning nature.

The table below lists the factors that lead to imbalance in Vata types, with recommendations that will help keep them balanced:

CAUSES OF IMBALANCE	
Overstimulation	Too many choices
Overexertion	Negative emotions
Irregular routine	Stressful situations
Exposure to cold and/or windy weather	Unpleasant interactions with others
Excessive travel	

cont. on next page

SIGNS OF IMBALANCE	
Hyperactivity	Restless
Easily distracted	High strung
Overly emotional	Forgetful
Anxious	Poor digestion
Nervous	Constipation
Fearful	Irregular appetite
Lonely	Spacey
Quickly changing moods	

RECOMMENDATIONS	
Establish and maintain a daily routine	Encourage naps to recharge physically and emotionally
Protect from cold, windy weather (hats are a must!)	Provide healthy and delicious snacks
Reduce excessive stimulation	Avoid inappropriate TV shows or video games
Help plan and make goals	Maintain a fixed bedtime routine
Guard against fatigue	Minimize the number of choices
Encourage focused activities	Emphasize creative activities

PITTA BODY TYPE

Pitta is *fire*—digestion, body heat, mental brilliance, physical strength, passion, and temper. Pitta is like the summer sun: hot, bright, and powerful. Pitta children are dynamic and reactive, and often possess brilliant intellects and warm emotions. Pittas love to solve problems, make decisions, and work toward specific goals.

Physically, Pittas tend to have a medium build. It may seem like a cliché, but Pittas often do have reddish hair, ruddy skin, and freckles. Pitta children are usually physically strong and resilient. Because they have lots of energy and are quite focused, Pitta types are often good athletes. In fact, they generally require a lot of physical activity to absorb their great energy. Their Achilles' heel is that their brain and physiology can quickly become agitated and imbalanced by two simple things: *not eating on time* and *overheating.*

Pitta types usually have strong appetites. Because of their excellent digestive power, coupled with their inclination toward vigorous activity, they need to eat ample meals and to *eat on time.* If the mealtime is delayed, or if they miss a meal entirely, their physiology will cause them to be impatient and irritable; they may even be irrationally angry. This is an especially important consideration at lunch. Since noon is when the digestive power is at its peak, it's ideal to give your Pitta child lunch as close to noon as possible. And if you're headed out for an extended shopping excursion, be sure to pack plenty of snacks and cooling drinks so you don't end up dealing with a temper tantrum in the middle of the mall.

Hot spices like peppers and chilies aggravate and imbalance Pittas, though they often enjoy the taste. Since these spices will overheat both the mind and the body—causing temper tantrums and heartburn, respectively—it's important to help your Pitta child favor cooling liquids and food.

Pitta types—and we can hardly emphasize this enough—become easily overheated, especially in the summer. Pittas generally want their sweaters off and the AC on cold, much to the distress of their Vata friends and relations. Keep your Pitta kids out of the hot summer sun; you will soon know all the shady spots in nearby playgrounds.

Swimming and skiing are great sports for Pittas, vigorous but cooling. If your Pittas' love of precision lures them to tennis, golf, or baseball, encourage them to wear a hat and move out of the sun when they're not actually playing. And don't forget sunglasses and sunscreen, because their eyes and skin are especially sensitive to the sun. Pitta children will usually drink moderate amounts of water, but if they become over-heated or are playing in the sun, they will need more in order to cool down and rehydrate.

Pitta children find it much easier to go to sleep than Vatas do. They enjoy physical activity and, if they have been busy during the day, should fall asleep quite easily. The only prob-lem may be that they want to figure out how the entire uni-verse works before they close their eyes. So stop any intense TV, games, and schoolwork well before bedtime, or they may wake up full of energy in the middle of the night. One tech-nique that works well is to tell the Pitta child a long, involved, tedious bedtime story in which almost nothing happens. This captures their attention but gives nothing for their lively mind to engage with, so they can settle down to sleep.

Pitta toddlers often give up their naps before other children do: the world is so fascinating—who wants to sleep in the middle of the day? They'll generally make up for any missed rest by sleeping deeper and longer at night. If the lack of a nap causes concern at child care, you might suggest that your Pitta child look at picture books or quietly work on a puzzle while the other children nap.

The brilliant Pitta nature shows clearly in their speech. Pitta babies take an average time learning to talk, but when they do, their words are clear and decisive. Or, with their love of perfection, they may be reluctant to speak until they're sure they can do it exactly right. Thus they start talking late but amaze you with the ideas they then express. When they start school and learn to write, the stories they come up with are often far ahead of their age group.

Pittas can be excellent problem solvers. They love to test their ingenuity, and stay focused until they figure it all out. This means that school is generally easy for them, as long as their teachers can keep the bright Pitta intellect occupied and challenged. If you want to keep your young Pitta engaged, puzzles and mazes will work better than coloring books and stickers. A bored Pitta child can be hard to handle when he starts looking for something to occupy that energetic and inquisitive little mind.

Pittas tend to be naturally competitive, which helps them perform well in school, sports, and other competitions. But their focus on winning can turn into fiery aggression. People are drawn to a *balanced* Pitta's warm nature, which, along with the Pitta's love of competition, often makes them natural leaders. Pitta kids love to take charge of situations and may become upset or demanding if they are not given control. Not only are Pittas competitive, they also tend to think that they know the perfect way to do things.

This table shows some of the factors that lead to imbalance in Pitta types, with recommendations to promote balance:

CAUSES OF IMBALANCE	
Overheating	Hot spices such as chilies
Not eating on time	Negative emotions
Not drinking enough water	Violent video games or Internet before bed
Overly competitive or aggressive situations	

SIGNS OF IMBALANCE	
Irritable	Intense hunger
Angry	Excessive thirst
Impatient	Sensitivity to spicy and/or fried foods, with indigestion and/or heartburn
Critical	
Jealous	Excessive sweating
Hostility	Temper tantrum
Obsessive-compulsive behaviors	

cont. on next page

RECOMMENDATIONS	
Make sure meals are on time, especially lunch	Lots of physical activity during the day
Prevent overheating and immediately help them cool off with a cool drink	Try to avoid violent games or TV shows several hours before going to bed
Keep them well hydrated	On hot days keep the air-conditioning on; on mild days keep the windows open
Never serve foods with "hot" spices	Do not overdress a Pitta child

KAPHA BODY TYPE

Kapha embodies *solidity*—bones and muscles, fat and sinews. Kapha is like the earth in early spring: cool and moist, solid, and a bit heavy. Kapha children are steady and strong, physically, mentally, and emotionally. They also have the sweetness of spring, and like spring, they can be slow to get going, but you can count on them to show up eventually.

Physically, Kaphas are generally strong with excellent stamina. They have a sturdy build, not necessarily large, but solid. Kapha children usually enjoy lots of physical activity—once you get them going, which may be a challenge. They embody Newton's First Law: a body at rest tends to stay at rest; a body in motion tends to stay in motion. But Kaphas *need* physical activity or they tend to become sluggish, so include periods of regular activity and exercise in their routine—preferably outdoors. Encourage them to join sports teams to keep them lively, socially as well as physically. They should do well at sports that require stamina, such as basketball and soccer, and those that require strength, such as wrestling.

Kaphas are not nearly as bothered by wind and sun as their Vata and Pitta friends are, but they are uncomfortable, and their health is vulnerable, in humid and damp weather. Help them stay in balance with a dehumidifier in the summer and hot tea in the winter.

Sleep is a Kapha's best friend. Kaphas fall asleep easily and have a far better chance of sleeping through the night than other kids do. The only problem you might have is getting them going in the morning. They usually continue with naps a little later than their friends do. (Try not to gloat over how quickly you can settle your little Kapha at nap time.)

Kapha children have strong appetites, but, unlike Pittas, they can eat late or miss a meal without problems. They really enjoy food, so you have to be alert so they don't overeat. Their love of food is exacerbated by their slow metabolism, so they easily gain weight. If they overload their digestive system with heavy fried foods and sweets, they can become congested, with a stuffy nose and wet cough. Encourage your Kapha child to eat lighter foods: wraps instead of burgers, chocolate-dipped strawberries instead of chocolate cake. Kaphas tend to be "foodies." If you're having trouble getting them out of bed, try motivating them by describing the delicious breakfast that is waiting for them. Better yet, if there is time, invite them into the kitchen to help prepare a scrumptious treat.

The most outstanding characteristic of a well-balanced Kapha child is steadiness. However, this very steadiness can slow them down because they do each part of a task so deliberately and methodically. A Kapha child is going to take a lot longer to put on socks, shoes, and a coat than their Pitta and Vata siblings, so get your Kapha started earlier.

Decision making is no different. They go over each choice systematically, scrutinizing all the possibilities. So, like Vatas, but for completely different reasons, they do better with fewer choices. Once they make their decision, it's the same story of immovability—it may take a charging elephant to persuade them to change their mind.

Mentally, Kaphas are steady, patient, thoughtful, and reliable. They tend to be methodical and slow in their learning style—slow to learn but *even slower to forget*! Kaphas learn most easily by doing; words, whether spoken or written, are too abstract, so they make little impression. So instead of talking or having the Kapha child read, provide *activities* for them to explore new concepts. The child with a concrete Kapha mind learns best if he can move it around or write about it: Unifix Cubes to learn subtraction, experiments in a chemistry lab, trying different knots when setting up a camping tent. They also need to do things *step by step*. A Pitta child may be able to remember and implement a list of instructions, but with Kaphas you need to tell them one thing and have them do it before you go on to the next.

Emotionally, Kaphas are generally sweet and compassionate. They are easygoing, much less disturbed by changes in their physical or social environment than other types. It's rare for Kaphas to become angry or frustrated. But if they don't have enough stimulation, their sedentary nature may lead them to become increasingly withdrawn. A Kapha who is out of balance is unlikely to do much, if anything, that requires effort. Left to themselves, this can spiral down into lethargy and depression. To lighten up an overly Kapha state, get them moving, put them in fun social situations, add more fresh fruit and crisp veggies to their diet. You might accomplish all three of these at once, for example, by inviting them to walk with you to a local market to pick out fresh produce.

Socially, Kaphas are generally loyal and supportive to others. Because they are so stable and impervious to changes around them, they rarely become overwhelmed and are usually good natured. When everyone around them is getting angry, anxious, and stressed, Kaphas feel stable and maintain their sense of humor. They can keep their heads in an emergency and may very well become the person everyone depends on when things get tough. When out of balance, however, Kaphas can become possessive because they don't want change—they want that person (or toy or favorite dress) to be with them forever.

Kapha types love having a stable routine. As with everything else, Kaphas need plenty of time to adapt to changes and disruptions. For example, tell them about a Thanksgiving trip to Grandma and Grandpa's well in advance. Make it concrete to them by showing them pictures of the cousins they'll meet there, the yard they'll play in, the house where you grew up. And while they love routine, they need to be stimulated and to get away from their set patterns. You and your Kapha child will do fine as long as you remember that they usually require extra motivation, stimulation, and time for any task.

This table lists some of the factors that lead to Kapha imbalance, with recommendations for steadying Kapha types:

CAUSES OF IMBALANCE	
Excessive sleep	Overeating
Too little activity	Exposure to excessively hot, humid weather
Lack of mental stimulation	
Lack of regular exercise	Exposure to cold, damp weather

cont. on next page

SIGNS OF IMBALANCE	
Stubborn	Sad
Depressed	Withdrawn
Lethargic	Excess mucus
Lazy	Weight gain
RECOMMENDATIONS	
Keep them mentally and physically stimulated	If it is too hot and humid move them to a dehumidified and cooler environment
Include periods of regular outdoor activity and exercise in their routine	In damp and cold weather offer them a warm drink and move them into a warm, dry environment
Try not to allow them to overeat: light meals are best	Give them time to adapt to a new decision
Allow them extra time to do everything	

BRAIN/BODY TYPES: EXTENSION OF THE TRADITIONAL AYURVEDIC MODEL

One area that has not yet been fully investigated by science is the relationship between the Ayurvedic types and brain functioning. Brain function underlies and drives all our thinking and action, so each of the different Ayurvedic mind/body types should show a distinctive pattern of brain functioning. This is an area that we are currently investigating. The Ayurvedic mind/body types can give us insight into how the brain functions, and neuroscience can help us understand the details of the Ayurvedic mind/body types. We've developed a theoretical model and are conducting research to test that model. We are particularly focusing on the executive system, located in the frontal lobes of the brain. This is the system that controls the brain's "higher" functions:

- interpreting information that comes in through the senses
- focusing attention
- controlling emotional impulses
- making decisions
- creating long-term plans

We suggest that in the Vata type, this system processes information very quickly and also tends to switch attention very rapidly. Because this type has more pieces of information to consider in any situation, and has trouble inhibiting emotional reactions, the Vata brain can be inundated by outside stimuli, disallowing focused attention, which leads to the possibility of mistakes. *This would explain why the Vata brain/ body type learns quickly yet can also become overwhelmed with too much information.*

In the Pitta brain/body type, we would predict that the brain's executive system processes information at a moderate to high rate, while at the same time focusing on details. Even with this great ability to focus, *the Pitta type sometimes cannot inhibit strong emotional impulses, particularly anger.*

The Kapha brain/body type processes information more slowly, but it is extremely reliable and accurate. *Consequently, Kaphas are slow learners, but at the same time their thinking is very methodical and steady.* The Kapha brain is also generally quite good at controlling the emotional centers. They are also the most emotionally stable type.

The massive reorganization of the brain during childhood will affect each body type differently depending on *which* brain areas are used most frequently, and *when* each brain area develops.

HOW TO IDENTIFY BRAIN/BODY TYPES

You may have already guessed your child's brain/body type from the descriptions above. And the simple quiz below will help you identify the brain/body type of everyone in your family. *Identifying brain/body types is your first step in learning how to deal with your child's natural tendencies, strengths, and weaknesses, and your own.*

This short quiz will give you enough information to begin using the Dharma Parenting tools. You will also find a more detailed quiz at **www.dharmaparenting.com**. This quiz gives a much more comprehensive summary of the particular mental, physiological, and behavioral characteristics associated with each type. In chapter 9 we introduce the traditional Ayurvedic method of determining brain/body type, the technique of self-pulse diagnosis.

BRAIN/BODY TYPE QUIZ

Vata Brain/Body Type

1. Light sleeper who has difficulty falling asleep

Strongly Disagree / Strongly Agree
[1]   [2]   [3]   [4]   [5]

2. Irregular appetite

Strongly Disagree / Strongly Agree
[1]   [2]   [3]   [4]   [5]

3. Learns quickly but forgets quickly

Strongly Disagree / Strongly Agree
[1]   [2]   [3]   [4]   [5]

4. Easily becomes overstimulated

Strongly Disagree / Strongly Agree
[1]   [2]   [3]   [4]   [5]

5. Does not tolerate cold weather very well

Strongly Disagree / Strongly Agree
[1]   [2]   [3]   [4]   [5]

6. Lots of physical energy but a sprinter rather than a marathoner

Strongly Disagree / Strongly Agree
[1]   [2]   [3]   [4]   [5]

7. Speech is energetic, with frequent changes in topic

Strongly Disagree / Strongly Agree
[1]   [2]   [3]   [4]   [5]

8. Becomes anxious and worried when under stress

Strongly Disagree / Strongly Agree
[1]   [2]   [3]   [4]   [5]

VATA SCORE
(Total your responses)   _____

Pitta Brain/Body Type

1. Gets overheated easily

Strongly Disagree / Strongly Agree
[1]   [2]   [3]   [4]   [5]

2. Reacts very strongly if challenged

Strongly Disagree / Strongly Agree
[1]   [2]   [3]   [4]   [5]

3. Gets irritated if meals are delayed

Strongly Disagree / Strongly Agree
[1]   [2]   [3]   [4]   [5]

4. Good at physical activity

Strongly Disagree / Strongly Agree
[1]   [2]   [3]   [4]   [5]

5. Strong appetite

Strongly Disagree / Strongly Agree
[1]   [2]   [3]   [4]   [5]

6. Good sleeper but may have
trouble falling asleep if
absorbed in some activity

Strongly Disagree / Strongly Agree
[1]   [2]   [3]   [4]   [5]

7. Speech can be precise and
articulate

Strongly Disagree / Strongly Agree
[1]   [2]   [3]   [4]   [5]

8. Becomes irritable and/or angry
under stress

Strongly Disagree / Strongly Agree
[1]   [2]   [3]   [4]   [5]

PITTA SCORE
(Total your responses)

_____

Kapha Brain/Body Type

1. Eats slowly

Strongly Disagree / Strongly Agree
[1]   [2]   [3]   [4]   [5]

2. Falls asleep easily but has a
hard time waking up

Strongly Disagree / Strongly Agree
[1]   [2]   [3]   [4]   [5]

3. Steady, stable temperament

Strongly Disagree / Strongly Agree
[1]   [2]   [3]   [4]   [5]

4. Doesn't mind not eating on
time

Strongly Disagree / Strongly Agree
[1]   [2]   [3]   [4]   [5]

5. Slow to learn but rarely forgets

Strongly Disagree / Strongly Agree
[1]   [2]   [3]   [4]   [5]

6. Good physical strength and
stamina

Strongly Disagree / Strongly Agree
[1]   [2]   [3]   [4]   [5]

7. Speech is slow and thoughtful

Strongly Disagree / Strongly Agree
[1]   [2]   [3]   [4]   [5]

8. Becomes possessive under
stress

Strongly Disagree / Strongly Agree
[1]   [2]   [3]   [4]   [5]

KAPHA SCORE
(Total your responses)

_____

NOTE FROM MOM

BRAIN/BODY TYPES FOR KIDS

Use your child's favorite storybook characters to teach your young ones about brain/body types:

Winnie-the-Pooh is a classic Kapha brain/body type: cheerful, chubby, compassionate, and sometimes a bit slow. Interestingly enough, his favorite food is honey, which Ayurveda extols as the ideal food to keep Kapha in balance!

Piglet and **Tigger** are typical Vata brain/body types: Piglet is small and often anxious or excited. Tigger is long and lanky and never, ever stops moving.

Rabbit is clearly a Pitta brain/body type: he bustles around taking charge of everything and everyone, and always knows best.

Eeyore is an unbalanced Kapha brain/body type: he is moody and depressed and grumpy, and moves very slowly. (A little of Pooh's honey might help him get back in balance.)

If you find that the quiz scores are high for any two different brain/body types, it simply means that the person is *a combination of types*, which is the case for most of us. For example, if your sturdy redheaded son has a strong appetite and becomes overheated easily yet at the same time he's very even tempered and slower to learn—he is likely a Pitta-Kapha type. For simplicity, we are focusing only on the three main brain/body types, Vata, Pitta, and Kapha, in this book, since one type tends to predominate in our physiology and behavior.

There is no one brain/body type that is better or more favorable than another. Each of the types, alone or in combination, is equally desirable *when it is in balance.* Each person can give a unique gift to the world and the key phrase here is "in balance." Armed with knowledge of your family's brain/body types, you can easily learn strategies to keep everyone in your family in balance. This, in turn, will support everyone's mental and physical health, comfort, success, and happiness. The more balanced each person becomes, the more their unique brilliance will radiate and the happier they will be.

COMPARISON TABLE OF RECOMMENDATIONS

The table below gives recommendations for diet and behavior in the first column. The smiley faces in the cells indicate which of the seven different brain/body types (which include combination types) should follow each recommendation. For example, the first recommendation, "Get extra rest," is critical for anyone with Vata as part of their brain/body type, especially if Vata predominates.

Copy the table below, or go to our website (**www.dharma parenting.com**) and print it out from there. If your kids are old enough, each one can take the quiz to figure out their own brain/body type. In either case, it will help to use a colored marker to highlight all the recommendations that apply to each type.

Look carefully at the different recommendations for each family member. For example, one child might be a Pitta type who requires air-conditioning to stay cool, while you (or another child) may be a Vata type who needs the heat on to be comfortable. No wonder you can't agree about the thermostat setting! With this insight, you can make adjustments to accommodate everyone. Your Pitta child can wear cooler clothing, and Vatas can wear a cozy sweater. As we've said before and will probably say again, knowing your child's brain/body type is the first tool of Dharma Parenting, because it provides the basis for understanding the different needs and tendencies of each member of your family.

RECOMMENDATION	VATA	PITTA	KAPHA	VATA/ PITTA	VATA/ KAPHA	PITTA/ KAPHA	VATA/ PITTA/ KAPHA
Get extra rest	☺			☺	☺		☺
Avoid caffeine after 11:00 a.m.	☺			☺			
Always keep warm (wear a hat)	☺						
Post a daily schedule for yourself according to priority	☺						☺
Accomplish your highest priorities first	☺						
Wind down before going to bed	☺			☺	☺		
Eat a good-sized meal on time		☺		☺		☺	☺
Don't get overheated		☺		☺		☺	
Avoid spicy foods		☺		☺			
Drink lots of liquids but avoid caffeine		☺					☺

cont. on next page

RECOMMENDATION	VATA	PITTA	KAPHA	VATA/ PITTA	VATA/ KAPHA	PITTA/ KAPHA	VATA/ PITTA/ KAPHA
Take a cooling-off period whenever you feel stressed		☺					
Resist overeating			☺		☺	☺	
Exercise daily			☺		☺	☺	☺
If you feel depressed, communicate with friends, family, or a professional			☺			☺	

Now that everyone has colored in their recommendations, your family may want to discuss how all the different recommendations overlap and contrast. Then you can post the table on your refrigerator as a reminder that different brain/body types structure your family dynamics!

NOTE FROM MOM

Brain/body types are not labels to excuse bad behavior *or* to criticize how a child responds to challenges. A Vata type will see the world very differently from a Pitta or a Kapha type. However, the differences can complement each other. Every child will bring his own point of view to enrich the situation. It is like many colored threads woven together to create a beautiful cloth.

CHAPTER 2

WHEN BRAIN/BODY TYPES COLLIDE

HOME IS WHERE YOUR CHILD first learns how to get along with others. Each new sibling changes your child's world, so it's extremely useful to understand *how different brain/body types interact*. Sit a Kapha and a Pitta type in front of a plate of spicy nachos. The spicy food will enliven the Kapha, but it will badly imbalance the Pitta. Pittas, especially, may thrive on physical competition, but a Vata child can be emotionally and physically overwhelmed in competitive situations. This may be extremely hard for a Pitta brain/body type parent to comprehend and sympathize with.

Problems between family members or among friends are very often a collision of the natural tendencies of brain/body types. This explains why some kids (and adults) seem completely unable to see another's point of view, and why it's hard for you to understand one of your children when it's so easy to relate to another. The knowledge of brain/body types helps you comprehend and resolve such situations, giving you concrete steps to diminish conflict and smooth the sharp edges of differences. More important, understanding that different brain/body types have different preferences and needs *built into their physiology* will help your children become more tolerant and learn to resolve their own differences: "Oh, he's not being slow just to make me mad, that's just his brain/body type!" or "Of course my sister never waits for me, she can't stay still and always has to run on ahead." Best of all: "The reason I'm slower (or more freckled, or smaller) than my friends is because that's how I'm made; it doesn't make them any better than me."

PLAYING WITH SIBLINGS AND FRIENDS

Imagine walking into a prekindergarten classroom, where groups of children are playing together. Some are sitting at small tables and chairs, working on a puzzle. Others play with Lego.

Another group is on the jungle gym, and they catch your attention because they're very loud. One child is at the top. Apparently he's "king of the mountain," and doesn't let any of the other kids up there. As more of them try to reach the top, he gets louder. Soon some of them are wrestling on the jungle gym and falling to the padded mat below.

Yet another group is sitting on soft, comfy chairs in a quiet area, with shelves of brightly colored picture books. The teacher is reading to a few children. Others are looking at books even if they can't read. Some kids are intently focused on the reading, while some sit and listen for a while and then run off to do something else.

Some kids are playing dress up. Two or three are picking out what they want to wear. A third is putting on a big bonnet and begins to narrate a fantasy in which everyone has a part. They're all talking excitedly.

The last group is sitting in the sandbox, playing with trucks. No one is talking very much but they all have smiles on their faces. They stay in the sandbox for the whole time you're there, happily building roads for their cars and trucks.

Children gather naturally into such separate groups because they share similar brain/body types. They get together to engage in the same activities because that's what they naturally want to do—be quiet, create a fantasy world, or compete. Let's consider the three main brain/body types in more detail.

VATA CHILDREN

The Vata children will probably be the ones playing dress up. They often opt for artistic activity (dance, theater, crafts, drawing, or painting) and admire what their friends create. Though they're naturally very social and enjoy each other's company, problems arise when Vatas go out of balance, which can happen easily with this very volatile brain/body type. Their love of movement and lack of focus can escalate into hyperactivity, and they can suddenly become overtired, which increases their tendency toward anxiety or fear. None of this supports a fun, coherent playdate. If one Vata child begins to feel tired and out of balance, it's important to monitor the situation closely since harmony is unlikely to last long.

In a family situation, older Vata brothers and sisters are

often very good company for your Vata toddler. They are naturally inventive, and if they're in good balance, they will work together to create a fun playtime out of whatever they can find.

When Vata children reach the teenage or young adult years, they're likely to be drawn to the company of other Vata friends who share their creative expressions. They will be best friends or best partners until one child goes out of balance (perhaps one of them happens to have a good amount of Pitta), at which point *both* can become emotional and irrational. This is a signal for them to take a break to recover, rebalance, and get grounded again. It will help Vata adolescents or teens to thoroughly understand their brain/body type so they know exactly what it is that puts them out of balance and what can help them regain equilibrium. Since Vatas forget so easily, you may have to find creative ways to explain the basic principles again and again until with experience they are firmly planted in your child's mind.

PITTA CHILDREN

In the pre-K classroom, one group of Pitta kids is working on the puzzle; another is playing on the jungle gym. Pittas are drawn to puzzles because they love to use their brilliant intellects. The Pittas on the jungle gym are the feistier, spirited Pittas who naturally like to have their own way. When they are balanced, Pittas are happy to play together and will enjoy each other's company, often working together to reach a common goal. But if they are out of balance, be prepared for a toddler match-off that can quickly result in hitting or crying. Both Pittas want to be in charge, and because each is sure he is right, their fiery Pitta tempers will flare.

In your family, if a Pitta toddler plays with an older Pitta brother or sister, you must make very sure that the older Pitta siblings are kind to the younger child. When older Pitta children are well balanced, they can be very responsible, but you have to make sure that these *natural commanders* don't boss the little one too much, and that they're not enforcing the rules too harshly.

You will notice that when Pittas participate in any situation with other Pittas, they frequently compete with each other. They revel in all types of sports and games—physical, board, or electronic. They love challenges and tests of their mental abilities, and they also enjoy passionate conversation. You might think they're arguing and becoming too emotional or angry, especially if you're a Vata type, but when you ask them how they're doing, if they are in good balance, they'll almost certainly look up and say, "Great!" The reality is that they're enjoying the competition and mental sparring.

During the teen and young adult years, Pitta with Pitta is an excellent combination for siblings, friends, and teammates. They have each other's backs and can work in harmony toward a common goal. When they're out of balance, however, the teamwork is lost, and they will argue and fight over even tiny issues as both struggle to be in charge.

KAPHA CHILDREN

In the pre-K classroom, the Kapha kids are the ones building roads in the sandbox. They're not running around; they're not talking nonstop. And they're really enjoying the simple power of trucking sand from place to place and building with it.

Kapha types are innately easygoing. They are slow to anger and tend to be supportive of others. How easy life can be—two happy Kapha children smiling at each other. Even if one of them goes out of balance, it's usually not hard to cheer him up as long as the other Kapha toddler remains content and relaxed.

In a family situation, if a Kapha toddler is playing with an older Kapha brother or sister, it's an almost ideal combination, and you'll probably see lots of hugging and sweetness. When Kapha children are out of balance, though, you need to watch for interactions that involve their being too possessive or too withdrawn.

As they become teenagers or young adults, two Kaphas make marvelous siblings or friends—happy, easygoing, and totally comfortable with each other. Out of balance, however, they really need your help to keep them from pulling away from each other. They don't express their feelings easily, so they can become depressed and stagnant, unwilling or unable to take the chance or make the effort to bridge the gap that has grown between them.

INTERACTIONS BETWEEN BRAIN/BODY TYPES

Any group of children will include a variety of different brain/body types. These mixes lead to dynamic interactions and often work well, with everyone's natural tendencies being balanced in the group. But they can also be tricky, so you need to simply be aware of each of the different brain/body types.

VATA CHILD WITH PITTA CHILD

As long as both are in good balance, the Vata-Pitta combination works well. When they're young, they will tend to both mind their own business and have a jolly time. A slightly older

Vata child will be full of ideas and suggest new things to do every other minute. The Pitta child loves the challenge of taking one idea to completion—and then, and only then, considers what to do next.

When they're both out of balance, however, the Pitta child can grow impatient and irritable, while the Vata child can be overly sensitive and demanding. Be prepared to intervene frequently to make sure that the Pitta child does not overpower the Vata child, and that the emotional Vata child does not drive the Pitta child mad. Vata is represented by wind and Pitta is represented by fire. Too much wind causes a fire to flare up, and when the flames become too high, everyone gets burned.

If your Vata toddler is playing with an older Pitta brother or sister who goes out of balance, a potentially explosive situation may develop, which could, at the very least, hurt the feelings of the Vata child. Both the age and the physical strength of the older child can easily overwhelm the sensitive Vata, so you have to create and enforce clear rules to protect the more delicate toddler.

During the teen or young adult years, when relationships between boys and girls begin to become serious, this combination can turn into an archetypical pairing of a strong Pitta male with a delicate Vata female—think prom king and queen. The Vata's creativity brings up new areas for the Pitta to master. Out of balance, however, this is a combination that can spell trouble, with the sensitive Vata's feelings being hurt and the Pitta becoming irritable or angry, and probably self-righteous.

VATA CHILD WITH KAPHA CHILD

The good-natured Kapha child can easily put up with the quickly moving, whimsical Vata. If the Kapha child is out of balance, however, he may be possessive or become upset by the rapidly changing nature of the Vata sibling or friend. An imbalanced Vata child will naturally become impatient and unhappy because he will not understand the slow steadiness of the Kapha. If the s-l-o-w Kapha and the quick Vata can't be reconciled, the best solution may be to give each his own space.

A Vata toddler playing with an older Kapha brother or sister should be a good combination if the older child is protective and kind to the little Vata sibling. But if the older Kapha child happens to be out of balance, he may be less accepting, and you will need to be alert and intervene before the situation sours.

In the teen or young adult years this combination can be a complementary blend of opposites. To return to our archetype, it's not unusual to see a small, young Vata woman walking arm in arm with a larger Kapha young man. The calm and steadiness of the Kapha male is a steadying anchor and a safe emotional haven for the Vata woman.

PITTA CHILD WITH KAPHA CHILD

A balanced Kapha child can usually put up with an energetic Pitta child. The Kapha child actually enjoys being "nudged" by a Pitta friend to get going, feeling it as a tickle, rather than a poke. The Kapha child is happier once engaged and moving, so the Pitta energy and drive may be just what's needed. But beware: If either of them is out of balance, everything can blow up. The Pitta child may overwhelm the Kapha child with fiery badgering, and the Kapha child may withdraw and completely freeze up.

A Pitta toddler playing with an older Kapha brother or sister is one of the best combinations. Even when the Pitta toddler is out of balance and a bit irritable, the situation can still be fairly comfortable because the Kapha's stability can absorb the Pitta's negativity and sweeten it. An imbalanced older Pitta, however, is unlikely to be able to be patient with a slower and less energetic Kapha toddler. On the other hand, the sweetness of the Kapha child may charm the older Pitta's sourness and the situation could resolve itself. The best solution might be to give each child his own space until both are balanced.

When this combination reaches the teen or college years, the pairing of Pitta and Kapha work well as a team, one providing dynamic energy while the other contributes steady power.

THE PARENT-CHILD RELATIONSHIP

You are, of course, a vital part of the equation. Most of us enter parenthood with our own hot buttons (whether we recognize them or not), which can be unintentionally pushed. Knowing your brain/body type, however, will help you understand why you have certain "buttons," and how to defuse them. And comparing your brain/body type with those of your children will help you figure out why you respond to them as you do, and vice versa. This knowledge will allow you to use your Dharma Parenting skills to accommodate brain/body type differences, because *knowing that each person is different by nature—rather than out of sheer contrariness—will really help you to be patient with everyone's quirks and needs.*

THE VATA PARENT

As a Vata parent, your strengths are your flexibility, your creativity, and your lightheartedness. When a problem arises, you can usually figure out several possible solutions to choose from. Your kids love how you sometimes whisk them off on spur-of-the-moment adventures. But Vata parents sometimes don't have enough stamina for the intense 24-7 focus and resolve that parenting requires. You may find your mind going in a million directions at once, your anxiety shooting through the roof, and your energy level dropping fast. This is why you, more than any other brain/body type, need to figure out how you can take a break, and settle your wild Vata physiology down, and generally reenergize and regroup. Maybe you can arrange for everyone in the house to take a period of quiet time, with Vata aromatherapy, soothing music, and comfy cushions to lie around on. And if you have learned Transcendental Meditation, be sure to find twenty minutes to do it, even if you have to wait until everyone else is in bed. TM is by far your most powerful tool to keep your Vata balanced so you're at your best.

Vata child with Vata parent. If you and your child are both Vata, you'll be in tune with each other from the start because your inclinations and interests are so similar. You're both quick-witted and have an innate ability, as well as the desire, to express yourselves, sometimes talking up a storm. You will love to create all sorts of arts and crafts projects together.

Because you may have already figured out some methods to help keep your own Vata in balance, you might instinctively know how to nurture your Vata child. For instance, you may have already learned that you have to dress warmly in cold weather, and you'll naturally dress your Vata child accordingly. From your own experience, you know very well that scary books or movies overexcite and upset Vata types. And you also know that when your Vata children come home from school, the first thing they need is a warm, tasty snack, plus some quiet time so they can settle down from all the activity and excitement of the day.

As your Vata child grows older, the two of you can share artistic endeavors, such as music, art, writing, or dance. You may even understand each other so well that you automatically complete each other's sentences. The downside of this simpatico relationship occurs when the Vata parent—that's you—becomes stressed or fatigued, and your unbalanced anxious "shadow side" takes over, impacting the emotional (and even the physical) stability of your highly sensitive child. Vata parents can easily become overwhelmed when pressures build and their schedule gets hectic. It's not that you're weak; it's simply part of your nature, a Vata characteristic. If you understand this Vata tendency, you'll be more likely to arrange for outside help and get as much extra rest as you can, especially during demanding periods.

Pitta child with Vata parent. A Pitta child can be very challenging for the Vata parent. You may find that the Pitta child's energy and more extreme needs overwhelm you, so use your flexibility and amazing creativity to find ways to keep your Pitta child engaged and focused. *Get extra help if you possibly can*—it will help to have an understanding partner and friends. If you can stay at least one step ahead of your intense Pitta child, things can be managed.

The situation becomes even more complicated as your Pitta child turns into a teenager. When they're in good balance, Pitta teens tend to organize their own lives, succeed in school and sports, and show strong leadership. But when they're out of balance, their excess energy and drive can lead to risky and even destructive behavior. When you, the Vata parent, are in good balance, you can be flexible, fun, and overflowing with ideas to help your Pitta teen move forward and fulfill his dreams. Pitta teens need to be challenged, and if they don't find enough challenge in school, sports, or other organized activities, they'll go out looking for it. Since their brains are far from being fully developed, their self-designed challenge may be foolish or even dangerous. If you're out of balance, your vacillating Vata attention and emotional strength may not be enough to rein in your Pitta teen's energy and inventiveness, and your teenager will have too much freedom.

Kapha child with Vata parent. A Kapha child makes parenting simple and sweet for Vatas (who might even be fooled into thinking that parenting is easy). Kapha babies often sleep through the night quickly, which, for Vata parents, is a gift from heaven. Your natural liveliness and creativity will keep your laid-back Kapha child stimulated and interested in new adventures. And you're always on the move and looking for new ways to engage your child in exciting activities, which is vital for their mental and physical well-being.

However, your Vata can also make you vulnerable, since you can be physically and emotionally delicate. You may become too tired and unfocused to be able to give your child the attention and direction he needs. And if your Kapha child becomes aggravated at the same time, he will withdraw and become inactive. The best solution, of course, is prevention. Pace yourself, stay rested, get extra help, maintain a firm schedule, and keep warm and grounded.

THE PITTA PARENT

As a Pitta parent, your strengths are your physical energy, warmth, organizational ability, and intelligence. Your lively intellect can stimulate your children's curiosity about the world, and your warm heart gives them a sense of security and being well loved. Of all three brain/body types, you're almost certainly the most proactive. Because you are good at (and enjoy) solving problems and planning ahead, you naturally visualize difficulties before they arise and figure out how to avoid them. But your Pitta focus may be *too* strong—you get so caught up in the task at hand that you can be unaware or even disregard the feelings of those around you, or you may overlook a family situation that needs your immediate attention, in favor of some interesting professional problem. And if your own Pitta becomes aggravated by overheating, delayed meals, spicy foods, or someone challenging your authority, the extra heat can set off explosions.

Of all types, you most need to keep your cool. Do not allow yourself to get hungry or thirsty. You can see that it aggravates your Pitta child, and of course, it does the same to you. Try to limit outdoor summer activities to the cool of the early morning or evening; if your child's T-ball game or tennis match is at noon, wear a hat, try for a seat in the shade, and keep your water bottle handy. Ice cream or a milkshake afterward is not only a treat but will help cool down your Pitta. Pitta aromatherapy, especially at night, can be very effective. If you know that you might be entering into a confrontation—negotiating with your teenager about prom night, for example—plan to do it only after a good meal when everyone is fed and rested, and provide cool drinks.

Vata child with Pitta parent. This can be a good combination during the first year when your Vata baby needs a lot of attention and, as a strong Pitta parent, you have stores of energy. Structure helps Vata babies, and Pitta parents are good at creating and maintaining structure. However, as your Vata child grows older you will quickly need to be alert for possible conflicts. Being Pitta, you have an entirely different physiology, nervous system, and personality. Pitta parents must be protective of their Vata child's more delicate physiology, and be much gentler with his emotions.

Pitta parents, with their dynamic and reactive nature, have to learn to truly *understand and empathize* with—*rather than dominate*—their Vata child. It may be that you speak too loudly or too harshly for your Vata child. And when you're frustrated, or trying to correct your child, your Pitta intensity may frighten your son or daughter without you being aware of it. Ask your child about this (the answer may surprise you). When you're talking things over or questioning your child, be sure to allow plenty of time for him to gather his thoughts and figure out how to explain the feelings involved. Children are naturally more scattered than adults, and Vata children more than other kids. Sometimes children have to just keep talking in order to figure out what they really want to say. Any impatience on your part will imbalance them even more, so you have to take the responsibility to cool your Pitta. You're the parent; be patient with your children, and listen to their thoughts and ideas.

As Vata kids pass through puberty, and especially during their teenage years, you need to be especially careful how you speak to them and how you treat them. If it sounds like we're suggesting that you wear psychological "kid gloves" with your Vata child, *you are absolutely right.* Kid-gloved carefulness is precisely how you want to behave for the good of your Vata child, whose nature is so different from and more sensitive than your own. Adolescents are in the process of figuring out for themselves how personal relationships work, so you want them to experience examples of patience, tolerance, and kindness. Researchers have found that thirteen-year-olds whose parents are overly dominating have trouble with personal relationships when they're eighteen and older. Put your attention on giving your sensitive Vata child a warm, cooperative, supportive role model so that she can develop those qualities in her friendships and attachments.

As a Pitta parent, you tend to expect quite a lot from your children because *you* are capable of discipline, orderliness, obedience, hard work, and high achievement. And it's hard for you to understand or tolerate "bad" or weak behavior. Self-righteousness—that deeply held confidence that your anger or approval is justified, as well as being good and useful for the child—is one of Pitta's "shadow sides," which can too easily appear when your Pitta becomes aggravated and imbalanced. When, however, your strong Pitta intellect is *balanced*, it can reassure you that your Vata child's skittishness, forgetfulness, and scattered thinking are *part of their nature, rather than the product of deliberate misbehavior on their part.* Work with your child to keep that delicate, lively Vata balanced. As the Pitta parent, you really are in charge, even when you're making allowances for the extreme difference of your Vata child's nature. Both your child's mental health and success in every endeavor is, to a large extent, in your capable hands. If you're balanced, the two of you will complement each other. Vata teens are imaginative and artistic, and you can enjoy a great deal of satisfaction and fun helping them channel their brilliant creativity toward excellence.

Pitta child with Pitta parent. A Pitta parent and Pitta child can be a great partnership when both are balanced. You share a love of structure and discipline, and you both possess high energy and physical and emotional resilience. Your lively Pitta intellect will find creative ways to stimulate your child's growing mind and body: games, excursions, and good talks together about how the world works. When your child starts school, you can enjoy his activities, from school projects to competitive sports. And your child will thrive on the attention you are able to give. As Pitta kids get older, try to think back to your own teenage years and remember how eager Pittas are to prove themselves and to exert their independence. Understand that in order to help them grow, you will need to become less involved in their projects, participating more on the level of appreciation and support, rather than giving suggestions (unless they ask for them).

If either one of you goes out of balance, a lot of heat and self-righteousness can be quickly generated. You both have strong opinions, and with your own built-in "hot button," arguments and power struggles may rapidly ensue. If you find yourself in the middle of an argument, and tempers are flaring, try to *stop*. Take a cooling-off period. Your angry Pitta child can cool off in his own room for a bit, and you can do the same in yours. When your emotional temperature returns to normal, offer cool drinks—and a hug. At this point, you may both be calm enough to work out your differences. But if either of you needs more time, try distraction; get your child interested in something else, a project or puzzle. Focusing that steamy Pitta intellect is very comforting and will help your son or daughter settle down. Maybe the two of you can try a new snack recipe—preferably something Pitta pacifying!

Brainstorming is another technique that may help you and your Pitta offspring come to agreement in an altercation. Give your child a marker to write down all the ideas the two of you come up with. This gives the Pitta intellect a neutral task to focus on instead of the argument. Set a timer for three to five minutes, and then think up as many solutions as you can. Nobody is allowed to comment on others' suggestions, no matter how silly or impossible they seem. After the timer rings, you both consider each idea and decide which ones are best. This is a great way to defuse a tense Pitta-Pitta confrontation.

Kapha child with Pitta parent. A Kapha child may be a complete mystery to the Pitta parent, whose natural speed is to move immediately, not in twenty minutes! You're a "doer" and a "finisher" and hate to leave anything less than fully done, and done well. Your Kapha child, on the other hand, is quite comfortable allowing you to blow by like a whirlwind, and then emerge from his room.

As a Pitta parent, you need to consciously adjust your speed and intensity in order to stay attuned to your Kapha child. The Kapha pace is naturally slower than yours, so you will need to learn patience—not a typical Pitta trait, but your strong intellect can help you understand the need for it. Kaphas also think much more concretely than you do—it's easy for you to imagine alternatives and their consequences, so you can make quick mental decisions. Your young Kapha, on the other hand, finds this far too abstract and does much better when he can make lists or draw pictures—better yet actually touch the different possibilities. For example, your Kapha child may not have an immediate answer if you ask, "What color sneakers do you want?" But if you're in the shoe store together, the child will love to consider each pair. You can speed the process along by limiting the choices; let your Kapha child pick from a limited number of pairs rather than from the entire store.

The Kapha child is more people oriented than goal oriented, and is, therefore, your direct opposite. Sometimes it might seem to you that your Kapha child isn't accomplishing much—but then you find yourself surprised by the warm praise of teachers and friends. Because you naturally function so differently, you must be careful not to project your priorities or your pace onto your Kapha child. Rather, take time to observe and allow your Kapha child to succeed in his own way. This may be an incredible challenge for you because you *really* like being in charge and getting things done, and you're good at it, but it's also fascinating to see how someone who functions so differently approaches problems and finds his own solutions.

THE KAPHA PARENT

As a Kapha parent, you provide stability, strength, and sweetness in your children's life. You are the bedrock, the foundation of their world. With your calm steadiness, you can structure and maintain a stable routine that provides a secure framework for their growth. And your stamina helps you ride out the ups and downs of parenting. But if you go beyond your limits of endurance, tiredness can drag that steadiness down into inertia, and your wonderful calmness down into passivity and emotional withdrawal. You need to carve some "off duty" time into your schedule in order for you to regroup and relax. While you may automatically opt for watching your favorite movie, remember that Kapha types are usually happier when making or moving. Crafts such as sewing or woodworking—useful projects requiring painstaking work—will probably make you feel more settled and satisfied than passive entertainment.

Kapha has a tendency to become sedentary, so keep yourself enlivened. Exercise is very important to keep your sturdy physiology from becoming sluggish and overweight. Can you make exercise a group activity? It doesn't have to be aerobics or calisthenics—a wild game of tag, a brisk walk, or shooting

hoops can get the family involved. Spicier, lighter foods—
think fruit instead of cake, tortilla chips and popcorn instead
of fries—will also help. Remember that even though Kaphas
are hard to get started, they are much more balanced, and
therefore happier, when they finally get moving. So try to talk
yourself ("trick" yourself if necessary) into starting an exercise
program or that upholstery project you've been thinking
about—it will help keep your Kapha brain/body type in good
balance, which will allow you to be a better parent.

Vata child with Kapha parent. The Kapha parent is a loving
and caring "earth mother" or father, who is nurturing and
happy—when in good balance. Your Vata child takes great
comfort from your steady, grounded Kapha nature. But if you
go out of balance, that wonderful stable support becomes
dulled down to unresponsiveness and lack of enthusiasm, and
the anxious Vata child will suffer. Kapha parents need their
rest, plus the loving support of their partners and friends, in
order to stay in balance.

As your Vata child becomes a teenager, a well-balanced
Kapha parent who is strong, dependable, and caring is exactly
what he needs. As a Kapha, you have the patience to deal with
the often unpredictable nature of Vata teens. For example, the
Vata child will often leave his room messy when, moving at
high speeds, he becomes immersed in one and then another
and another project. A balanced Kapha parent can handle this
easily, but an imbalanced Kapha parent will be too tired,
withdrawn, or laid-back. Your Vata teen will grow even more
chaotic if order is not restored. Stay in balance, Kapha parents: your Vata child desperately needs your stability, patience,
and support.

Pitta child with Kapha parent. A Pitta child can be a handful
for Kapha parents. Kapha parents are good at planning and

helping their kids maintain a stable routine, but the Pitta child can become frustrated that their parents aren't quick enough about changing the routine when something new and fascinating arises, *or quick enough about anything*. This may be magnified because you as a Kapha brain/body type probably enjoy and rely on the stability of a set routine, while your Pitta child is likely to want to be much more independent and self-determining.

The Kapha parent is usually calm—a definite plus in parenting—unless the lively intellect of that Pitta child of yours wants to argue every single point, partially for the fun of it, and partially because they want to lead. Once you realize that a pressing desire for change and discussing every possible option is part of the Pitta nature, your natural steadiness and patience will help you put up with these typical Pitta traits.

As your Pitta child grows older, life becomes even more challenging. Pitta teens like to be in charge and move things forward, and Pittas are often sure that they know the best solution to every situation. You may have to move faster than seems natural in order to keep up with—or ahead of—them if at all possible. As long as the Pitta teen is in good balance and moving in a positive direction, you can work together pretty easily. But if either you or your teenager goes out of balance, things fall apart. Fast. Your instinct may be to step back and take your time figuring out the situation, but this can allow your Pitta to move even further in the wrong direction. You need to be careful *not* to leave your Pitta teen to his own devices, which will be naturally one of his goals in life, even at this age. It's like they're born with "I can do it!" written indelibly across their foreheads.

Satisfy Pitta children's or teenagers' independent spirits by allowing them to make as many choices as they safely can;

knowing that if you trust them to make smaller decisions, they'll be more likely to work with you when making bigger decisions. Make sure that as a Kapha parent you keep yourself well rested and in balance—otherwise you may lose control of your strong-willed child. Keep yourself lively with exercise and plenty of rest. If you get too far out of balance, your Pitta child may feel that you're inattentive or cold toward them. If this escalates into feelings of hurt and abandonment, it's a signal for you to get professional outside help, and the sooner the better.

Kapha child with Kapha parent. From the very beginning, you will understand each other. Life can be simple and fulfilling when both parent and child are relaxed and content. You move at the same pace and enjoy the same lifestyle. Your main challenge may be to make sure you both stay lively and stimulated. Calm and laid-back is good, but sluggish and passive needs a jump start! This is why it's vital for both of you to get off the couch and go out and be challenged. Bike, walk, or run together. Better yet, build something together. And don't let winter weather stop you—go sledding, skating, shovel the sidewalk. Since Kaphas are hard to get moving, the toughest part will be to get yourself going first, and then get your Kapha child moving too. But once you both get started, watch out: you may enjoy it so much that you'll find it hard to stop on time!

One area to watch carefully is passive entertainment such as TV and video games. You *must* set an example by limiting your own downtime. One way to limit your children's computer access is to post a note every day: "To earn today's Internet password, do any two of the following chores. . . ." They'll be helping out—which is very satisfying for Kapha children, who like to complete concrete tasks—and at the same time learning that computer access isn't a given but a privilege.

It's hard to get even a balanced Kapha moving, and with too much Kapha it may seem nearly impossible. Too much Kapha means that you go from stable to immovable, from steady to depressed. Often the easiest way to begin to correct this is by purely physical means. Start with some Kapha aromatherapy: its spicy scent is *stimulating*. Then work on your diet: more hot spicy foods, more light dry foods, fewer cold foods such as ice cream, fewer heavy foods such as mashed potatoes and butter. Make a list of physical chores that really need doing—wash the windows, mow the lawn, run the dog, take a brisk walk to the grocery store. By energizing your physiology, you'll find that you start to feel livelier mentally as well: *change your physiology, change your brain!* Creating a new daily routine for yourself and your child that includes exercise or a new diet keeps both your Kapha brain/body types in good balance.

THE BIG PICTURE

Naturally, family life is not as simple as all that. More than one child increases the number of relationships that need to stay in balance. With one parent and two children, there are now three relationships instead of just one: the parent interacting with each child, plus the two children interacting. Add another child, and you've got six interactions! For example, you may find that you're not simply waiting for your slow Kapha preschooler to meticulously tie both shoes; at the same time you have to keep his Pitta older sister from getting upset because she's ready to leave, and you have to keep track of that

Vata toddler, who's running out the door ahead of everyone!

Add a second parent, and possibilities escalate further. Of course, this can be a real plus, because the two of you can complement and reinforce each other's natural parenting instincts. A Vata-Kapha parenting team, for example, provides both liveliness and calm steadiness for the family. Learning about brain/body types will help you realize that *your differences arise from your basic natures*—so you can be much more tolerant when you disagree about how to handle parenting. It will also help you consciously bring out each other's best parenting traits and compensate for any weaknesses. For example, suppose you're faced with the tricky task of setting curfew hours for your high school senior. The Vata parent can think of lots of possible solutions, while the Kapha parent can come up with a solid set of guidelines and make sure they are enforced. If a special situation arises, the Vata parent can convince the Kapha parent to make an exception. On their own, however, the Kapha parent might refuse to change the rules, even for prom night or the senior play cast party.

If you're a single parent, Dharma Parenting has your back. Most of the time, there isn't another adult around to help you figure out what's going on and how to deal with it. But understanding brain/body types will give you insights into your children's behavior and your own reactions to it: "To avoid those late-afternoon meltdowns, I need to keep my Pitta kids well fed and cool. And I have to watch my own impulsive Vata reactions and take time to think things through. Maybe when the kids get home from school and I get back from work, we can sit down and have a snack while we discuss how the day went and any issues we need to figure out. I'll be more rested then, and ready to cook dinner, and they can get started on homework."

As a single parent, you *know* how important it is to function at your best—and how *incredibly difficult* that can be. You are responsible for everything: earning the paycheck, housekeeping, keeping track of finances, and parenting. Make the parenting a little easier by using the tools and insights from Dharma Parenting and also by building a support group with family members and other single parents from work, friends, your child's school, or using community resources. One other piece of advice, which you've heard many times: Get enough rest. It might seem impossible—you already have way too many demands on your time! This is one reason that Transcendental Meditation is such a valuable parenting tool: In twenty minutes your mind becomes relaxed and clear, and your body unwinds and feels truly refreshed. You can fit TM into a slightly extended afternoon break at work, or on the way home if you take public transportation. Better yet, get your children interested too and enjoy a family meditation before dinner.

CHAPTER 3

THE SECOND TOOL OF DHARMA PARENTING:
Heal Yourself

Jason is a divorced dad with two young daughters he adores, five-year-old Hayley and seven-year-old Jana. They are only with him on weekends, from Friday evening through Monday morning, so he wants to spend as much time as he can with them. Jason's weekdays are incredibly taxing: he's a full-time delivery truck driver, and three months ago he started online courses to complete his master's degree in computer science. Classwork takes longer than he thought it would, and he studies late almost every night because he wants his weekends free to be with Hayley and Jana. By the time Friday rolls around, Jason is pretty exhausted. He's also feeling stressed because finances are tight, with child support and tuition payments.

When Jason took the online brain/body type quiz, he discovered that he is primarily Pitta but with a fair amount of Kapha. As time passes he begins to realize how much his fatigue is affecting his parent-

ing. He notices that he's often irritated instead of charmed by his girls' chatter and curiosity—why can't they be quiet for a little while and stop bothering him? As his fatigue deepens each week, he's starting to withdraw from them, participating less and less in their games and sometimes not responding at all. What can Jason do to fix this situation? How can he generate the energy and attention he knows he should be giving his daughters?

Monica is Hayley and Jana's mother, and every weekend she works three twelve-hour shifts as an emergency medical technician. On weekday mornings, she's the school nurse at Hayley's preschool. Theoretically, this is a great arrangement: she loves her EMT job and it pays most of the bills. And as the school nurse, she gets a substantial discount on Hayley's prekindergarten tuition; it's not a high-pressure job, and she has afternoons at home with Hayley. But overall, Monica is working fifty-six hours a week and she's starting to burn out. She finds that she doesn't stay focused very well—sometimes her girls ask why she's not paying attention to them. Her mind seems to be constantly caught up in problems. Monica doesn't need to take the brain/body quiz to figure out that she's a Vata type. And she is beginning to recognize that the anxiety that haunts her days and the churning mind that keeps her from falling asleep are both signs of aggravated Vata.

Effective parenting begins with effective parents. And a balanced, healthy, happy family begins with balanced, healthy, happy parents. But how is it possible to achieve this? How can a person manage a home, family, and job on only three or four hours of sleep? Even in-flight safety instructions tell us to put on our own oxygen mask before we help our children with theirs. "Attachment theory" in developmental psychology is in complete agreement with this instruction. And we know— from research on how children from various backgrounds grow into adults—that primary caregivers are critically important to a child's development. It's common sense, supported by a lot of careful research: when you—the parent—are awake, happy, sensitive, and strong, you will naturally nurture your children more easily and effectively, and they will feel loved and secure. If, however, you're fatigued, unhappy, insensitive, and inconsistent, you will probably tend to ignore them, and your children will feel unloved and insecure. Research has shown quite clearly that insecure children are more vulnerable to stress and have difficulty controlling anger and other negative emotions. Insecurity also affects the ability to think clearly, so insecure children tend to do poorly in school.

Whatever you do, do not ignore the signs of your own stress and fatigue, which can appear as depression, lack of energy, forgetfulness, irritability, insomnia, or just general unhappiness. It's important for you as a caring parent, and as a human being, to be rested, balanced, and whole. This is why the second step of Dharma Parenting is heal *yourself.*

KNOW YOUR BRAIN/BODY TYPE

By now you have completed the written quiz in chapter 1 or, even better, the more detailed online quiz at dharmaparenting.com, and you have discovered your child's brain/body type and your own. You've also read chapter 1, which gives you a list of basic recommendations to help each brain/body type stay in good balance. The next step is for you to actually *use* these valuable tools.

ASK FOR HELP

Jason is a natural problem solver, so once he admits to himself that he has a fatigue problem, he enjoys the challenge of figuring out how to fix it. He realizes that his schedule is just too packed, and he thinks if he could have half a day to rest and relax, it would be enough to keep him fresh. As it is, he's only getting five to six hours of sleep on weeknights, which is not enough. After thinking about it, Jason comes up with three possibilities:

- Maybe one of his daughters has a friend whose parents would like to trade off taking them for excursions on Saturday afternoons. If not, Jason will ask around both at work and in class to find parents with similar-aged girls who might like this arrangement.
- If this doesn't work, he could find a reliable high school student to take the girls out for half a day on weekends.
- Jason thinks he could rearrange his delivery route so it's more efficient, saving up to an hour a day. And since his boss is very supportive (he's the one who encouraged Jason to finish his degree), Jason thinks he can get permission to go home as soon as his route is finished and start studying an hour earlier on most days.

Jason's ex, Monica, is lucky because her mother lives nearby and is always sympathetic and ready to help. After their regular Wednesday night dinner at Grandma's house, Monica sends the girls to play in the living room and asks her mom to help figure out how she can get more rest. They decide that Grandma will have the girls at her house on Tuesday afternoons and evenings; she'll pick up Hayley at lunchtime and Jana after school, and bring them both home after dinner. Monica knows that the worst part of the week is Monday morning, when her EMT shift ends at 4:00 a.m. and her school job starts four hours later. Taking a hard look at her budget, she decides that if she's careful, she can afford to cut out her Sunday–Monday shift every other weekend. (She tries to convince the afternoon nurse at school to switch Tuesday afternoon for her Monday morning shift, but no luck.)

If you're feeling tired or stressed, you might consider Jason and Monica's example. Examine all your commitments and see where you can make adjustments. You don't have to do this alone—in fact, it's quite hard to do it by yourself. Never feel ashamed or shy to *ask for help when you need it*. You know that your children are important, *and so are you*. Many parents are in a similar predicament, so when you ask for their help, you can, in turn, relieve some of their load. Grandparents, aunts, and uncles all want the best for your children, and they often enjoy a chance to spend time with them. You may actually be doing them a kindness, too, when you ask for their help.

As single parents, Monica and Jason must look a little harder for support systems, but usually your partner is your first line of help. If you're both learning about brain/body types, it will be easier to recognize the characteristic signs when the other person needs a break: the Vata's anxiety or sleeplessness, the Pitta's irritability or anger, the Kapha's grumpiness or lethargy.

FATIGUE IS THE ENEMY

When we're tired, the first part of the brain to go off-line is our prefrontal cortex, which is the seat of executive processing—the "boss" of the brain. This is the part of the brain that distinguishes right from wrong, predicts future outcomes, controls social behavior, and makes plans toward goals. So with these important areas off-line, it's much harder for us to remember things, to plan, to master new tasks, to solve problems, and to deal with challenges.

Here's what lack of sleep does to our brain: When we're fatigued, the amygdala, which is the seat of all fears and phobias, fires 60 percent more often. At the same time, lack of sleep breaks the neural connections between this emotional system (the amygdala) and the prefrontal cortex, which is the part of the brain that judges how appropriate our actions are. The end result is that when we're tired we react too quickly to situations, rather than reflecting upon them. We can also become overwhelmed by problems and be unable to see creative solutions. Emotions may grip our mind, and we can't find a way out. Fatigue impairs both our decision making and our performance. Being exhausted leads to memory deficit, slower reaction time, and increased mistakes of all kinds. Research has revealed that people who work more than seventy hours a week function as though they are legally drunk.

So sleep deprivation is a *big* stress. Regardless of what's causing the sleep loss, it impairs brain functioning and contributes to cumulative wear and tear on the body. Chronic sleep deprivation decreases immune functioning and makes us more susceptible to colds and flus. It also increases sympathetic activity in our nervous system, creating the fight-or-flight response, so we become overemotional and irritable. Sleep deprivation also raises our blood pressure and elevates levels of both insulin and blood glucose.

About those middle-of-the-night wake-up calls: Our brain doesn't simply slow down during sleep; whole areas of the brain systematically switch off as we go to sleep and turn on again when we awaken. And when we wake up, our frontal lobes do not start functioning immediately. It takes time for them to wake up so that we're again able to plan, make decisions, and effectively direct our activity. This period between waking up and being able to think and plan even has a name, "sleep inertia." The impact of sleep inertia is greatest during the first three minutes after awakening, and though it dissipates after about seven minutes, its effects can still be detected up to two hours after waking. So be careful when you force yourself to wake up to respond to your crying child; your frontal areas are not yet active, so you don't want to attempt anything new or very complex.

GET MORE AND BETTER SLEEP

Clearly, the fact that you're overtired is seriously and immediately important. Not only are your health and sanity at stake, your child's welfare is too. *You've got to figure out a way to get more rest.*

Our friends Monica and Jason have adjusted their schedules so they now have time to get almost enough sleep every night. And since Jason has implemented the improved delivery schedule at work, he's getting home an hour earlier, and can get to bed an hour earlier. Being a Pitta-Kapha type, Jason generally has no problem falling asleep. With the extra rest, he's already feeling more alert and efficient, and is able to

spend less time on his schoolwork, which means he gets to bed
even earlier—in time for almost eight hours of sleep every
night. Instead of being caught in an endless spiral of fatigue,
he feels as if he's on a spiral of increasing alertness. On the
weekends, he's starting to get back his usual energy level and
is once again his girls' "best daddy."

As a Vata brain/body type, Monica has difficulty going to
sleep and staying asleep. Even though she went to all that
trouble to change her work schedule, she's still not feeling
rested. Whether it's a weekday with her daughters or a weekend of EMT work, by bedtime her mind is whirling and re-
sists settling into sleep.

Here are some steps Monica can take to help quiet her
mind at bedtime:

1. Set up a nighttime routine

   Monica needs to manage her kids' bedtime routine
   so that they're in bed and ready for sleep by 7:30 or 8:00
   p.m. This will give her the time her Vata brain *needs* to
   unwind before she goes to bed.

2. Begin the bedtime routine earlier

   A warm bath and quiet music will help begin the
   unwinding process that precedes sleep. And aromatherapy
   can often be amazingly effective at bedtime. (Monica
   would probably benefit from organic Calming Vata
   Aroma Oil, as well as one of several other sleep-promoting
   aromas.) Reading a soothing book—with no violence,
   no exciting ideas, just a calm and uplifting story—for a
   little while might also help her restless mind settle
   down.

3. Reduce caffeine consumption

In chapter 1, we mentioned that it's best for Vatas to be modest with their morning hit of caffeine and to avoid it entirely after 11:00 a.m. The research shows that even if you don't notice much effect, caffeine increases the average time it takes to fall asleep; it also increases the number of times you wake up during the night and decreases your total hours of sleep.

How on earth, Monica wonders, is she going to get through those long hours of EMT duty (not to mention Monday mornings) without caffeine? She eventually grasps that there's only one answer: *not to be so tired to begin with.* And she's figured out that she could be sleeping during her shift when she's not out on a call. Monica never used the EMTs' bunk room much while on duty because her mind wouldn't settle down and let her sleep; instead, it would keep busy with her laptop or her knitting. But after she found that aroma oil and a quiet book helped her sleep at night, she decided to try them at work. Her EMT team doesn't mind the smell of aroma oil in the bunk room—they need to settle down as much as she does—and now she manages to doze off between calls. On an occasional quiet shift, Monica may get as much as four to six hours of sleep.

At bedtime, it's important to allow your mind to settle down and *let go* so that you can gradually relax into sleep—but we know that this isn't always what happens. Again this is a situation in which Transcendental Meditation can be a "parent saver." Twenty minutes twice a day will calm your mind and relax your body so you can begin to have a profound night's sleep. TM is not a sleep aid—and the instruction is not to meditate right before bed—but the overall calming effect of daily Transcendental Meditation will allow you to settle down more easily at bedtime and improve the quality of both your day and your sleep.

EXERCISE

Everyone knows that exercise is essential for good health, and there are times when parenting automatically provides plenty of it. If your child is an infant, we promise that you won't have to worry about getting enough exercise for very long: once your little one starts to walk, you'll be running all over the house. Parenting also improves upper body strength. You start by picking up your infant and carrying him around every day; as the child gets a little heavier each week, you find yourself in training to become a champion weight lifter. Pretty soon you'll be running after your mini soccer player, which will provide aerobic exercise as well.

The fact is that everyone benefits from easy, repetitive exercise, preferably in fresh air. Walking is good not only for your body, but also for your brain. The human brain evolved while we were constantly moving hunter-gatherers, and neuroscience has found that our brain functions best while we are moving at 1.8 mph—an easy, comfortable walking pace. Exercise increases blood flow to our brain, so it makes sense that regular walking improves memory skills, learning ability, concentration, and abstract reasoning. Exercise actually changes the physical structure of our brain, creating more blood vessels and new brain cells.

Exercise also helps your body handle stress. Physical activity stimulates the physiology to produce more endorphins, those "feel-good" neurotransmitters in your brain. And while you're exercising, whether it's a game of tennis or a walk in the woods, you tend to focus on the activity and forget about the chaos everywhere else. Increased blood flow also helps wash away the stress chemicals in your blood. It's because of all this that exercise frequently improves the quality of your sleep.

Be sure to take your particular brain/body type into account when planning your exercise program. For example, as a Vata, Monica is enthusiastic about trying new programs or sports. And there are a lot of activities that are well suited to her quick bursts of energy and agile movement, including dance, yoga, water aerobics, and gentle cycling. But Monica doesn't have time to travel to a dance studio or pool, so a DVD for home use seems to be the best option. After narrowing her choices to Zumba and Pilates, she remembers that Vatas have a tendency to overdo things, so she decides on the less vigorous Pilates. The slower pace will allow her to check in with herself frequently and keep her from overexerting.

Jason also realizes that he needs to include regular exercise in his weekly schedule. Because Pittas are generally strong and love challenges, Jason would normally gravitate toward more demanding sports. But he already gets a physical workout with his delivery job and feels he needs a more fun, active sport. He is learning that he tends to get overheated and angry or irritated—and understands that his Pitta must be aggravated, so he decides on swimming. As an online student, Jason gets a discount at the college indoor pool, and on the weekends he can take his daughters and teach them to swim. (If they lived near the mountains, he might have chosen skiing.)

If you're a Kapha brain/body type, your strength and endurance suit you for strength training, as well as exercise programs such as aerobics or Zumba, and running sports such as soccer and basketball. The Kapha physiology is very stable, and exercise is vital to your being in balance—without it, your steadiness may deteriorate into inertia. It might take a lot of determination and self-discipline to get yourself moving, but *it's worth it*. Not only is it fun, but you'll enliven both your body and mind. Kaphas generally do well with a set routine, so figure out where exercise can fit into your schedule. Be consistent and it will be easier and easier to get moving.

YOGA

Yoga is different from physical exercise, because in addition to limbering the body, it calms the mind, helping to decrease anxiety and improve mood. Working on both the body and the mind, yoga can be a great stress buster. But, as with all types of exercise, it's important to tailor it carefully to your brain/body type.

If you're a Vata type, look for classes that incorporate the concept of flow. Too much vigorous movement will aggravate your Vata, while slower-paced classes will keep you calmer, and allow you to stay more aware of your body and avoid overdoing it. If your Vata goes out of balance, normally flexible joints may become a bit stiff, and in this case be especially careful not to strain—work up to that perfect pose over time.

If you're a Pitta type, your competitive nature may lead you to try perfecting difficult postures long before your spine is ready for it. Look for an instructor whose emphasis is on fun, dynamic, and improvisational classes—not only will this appeal to your Pitta nature, but a constantly changing yoga sequence will provide less opportunity for you to work yourself into knots trying to perfect each pose. And you probably want to avoid "hot yoga." A humid 104°F room will not help cool down the Pitta you're trying to balance.

If you're a Kapha type, more challenging yoga classes are for you. It's important for you to start off slowly, but your physical power and stamina will help you progress quickly. Look for classes and instructors that favor dynamic and vigorous sequences, as long as they're not too fast for your steady Kapha nature. If you're a little pudgy around the middle, yoga postures that require bending at the waist are recommended.

HOW TO DEAL WITH STRESS

In addition to dealing with their jobs and their relationship, Jason and Monica are also trying to cope with the various stresses that seem to be built into parenthood. Their weekly schedules reveal that they're both under great time pressure, working and studying over fifty hours a week. And both of them want to be loving, attentive, creative parents, which increases demands on their energy and inner resources. But now that they've started getting more rest and exercise, it's time for them to put attention on reducing their stress levels.

Challenge versus stress. It's important to distinguish between challenge and stress because the two are fundamentally different. Some people say that they need "stress" in order to function at their best and assert that they are more creative under "stress." What they're really talking about is the enhancing effect of *challenge*, rather than the debilitating effect of stress.

When we respond to a challenge, we tend to think and act at the upper limit of our abilities, drawing on our storehouse of mental and physical energy to generate creative solutions. As our brain responds to a challenge, it becomes flooded with a chemical called noradrenalin, which *speeds up* brain processing. Our sensory areas perceive more clearly and distinguish finer details. Our motor system is primed *to go*, and the frontal executive areas function faster. This is how *challenge* supports optimal performance.

If a challenge becomes too great, however, it initiates a stress response—that familiar fight-or-flight reaction that speeds our heart rate and tenses our muscles. Our body speeds up but our brain downshifts, turning off the frontal executive areas and switching to more primitive responses. We lose broad perspective entirely and experience tunnel vision, focusing on immediate details and missing the big picture. This response is appropriate and useful in an emergency. If the car starts skidding toward a ditch, for example, we don't need to consider our long-term goals; we need to focus sharply and respond immediately.

The problem is that chronic stress creates a *constant* fight-or-flight response, which keeps our executive brain areas turned off. This hinders our ability to see the big picture and make effective long-range plans. Stress also disrupts the functioning of the hypothalamus, the part of the brain that regulates many of the body's basic functions, such as hunger, heart rate, and hormone production. So stress affects both our conscious ability to make decisions and our body's ability to maintain internal balance. Researchers have found that college students smoke more cigarettes, drink more caffeinated drinks, eat fewer healthy foods, neglect commitments, and spend money more recklessly during finals week, when stress is high and the brain's executive centers go off-line.

Parenthood is always challenging. But challenge is fun and calls up our creative resources. If, however, that challenge becomes stress, we lose our ability to deal with even the normal demands of parenthood. We become irritable or make mistakes that add to our already long to-do list. Unrelieved stress can actually make us ill—with headaches, depression, ulcers, even asthma and heart disease.

How can we keep challenge from escalating into stress? And if we're feeling stressed, how can we boost our inner resources so it doesn't overwhelm us?

Remember, *fatigue is the enemy.* Fatigue makes *everything* worse. The fatigue from even a few nights of interrupted or inadequate sleep reduces frontal brain functioning. Grab extra rest whenever you can; it refreshes the brain so you can better handle stress.

When our children are babies and toddlers, we can expect to encounter more than just a few nights of sketchy sleep, so we're always vulnerable to stress. It gets easier when they start sleeping through the night, and when they start school some of the daytime pressure eases as well. You want to be careful to give yourself a little breathing room; don't pack your schedule too tightly. This is what happened to Monica: When Hayley started prekindergarten, Monica added on her job as school nurse. It helped the budget but escalated Monica's time pressure from challenging to stressful.

Mother Baby Program. Maharishi Ayurveda offers a Mother Baby Program that facilitates a smoother postpartum adjustment, allowing for more harmonious family relations and an enhanced quality of life after childbirth. For further information on the Mother Baby Program, as well as important advice for pregnant mothers, you can go to our website, or to www.gmdousa.org/health/mother-baby-program.html.

MEDITATION AND STRESS

Everybody knows that meditation helps us deal with stress. The tricky part is that not all meditation is the same, and each type of meditation has its own goals, its own procedure, and its own benefits. Fred summed this up in an important scientific paper that compares different types of meditation techniques, showing clearly that *each type produces different kinds of changes in the brain*. His paper lists three main categories of meditation procedure, each with different effects on the brain:

- Focused attention (including Zen, compassion, qigong, and vipassana): gamma (fast) EEG indicates that the brain is working hard.
- Open monitoring (including mindfulness and Kriya yoga): theta (slow) EEG indicates that the mind is following its own internal mental processes.
- Automatic self-transcending (including Transcendental Meditation): coherent alpha1 (foundational) EEG indicates that the mind is alert but quiet.

The first two types of meditation construct mental tools to help us cope with life. Generally speaking, focused attention meditations train the mind to concentrate more closely and for longer periods; and open monitoring meditations cultivate insight and awareness of what you are thinking and doing.

Automatic self-transcending meditations are fundamentally different because they do not involve thinking about something—rather, they allow the mind to settle down to a very quiet state while becoming more alert. The goal of Transcendental Meditation, which is in this third category, is not to develop a specific mental ability, such as improved concentration, but rather to improve the mind's basic functioning by making it more settled and alert. The word "transcend" means to *go beyond*, and when we *transcend* during TM we go beyond thoughts and categories—we are, in effect, stepping outside the boundaries of our problems. After our TM practice, we come back to our problems better able to see the big picture and find creative solutions.

You may want to try a focused attention or open monitoring technique if you feel that you need to improve your focus or become more aware of your thought processes. But if you want to improve your ability to think creatively and handle stress (as well as improving your health and vitality), we recommend Transcendental Meditation. We have both been practicing TM since college and have found it especially valuable when we were raising our families. We have researched how TM works, and its benefits, for most of our professional careers. Because we've experienced—personally and as researchers—how effective TM is, Dharma Parenting focuses exclusively on the Transcendental Meditation technique. Our preference is shared by professional organizations. For example, the American Heart Association has published a statement concluding that TM is the only meditation technique effective in reducing blood pressure. A Stanford University study evaluated 146 independent research studies and concluded that TM is twice as effective as other techniques for reducing stress and anxiety. The simple fact is that the experience of transcending changes the way our brain functions, giving us a broader perspective and a greater sense of self. Every morning we wake up fresher, with more energy. We are more conscious—indeed, *more awake*. This is why practicing TM for a few minutes twice a day helps us to effectively deal with stress: it rejuvenates both body and mind, and enhances our creative problem-solving ability.

SATISFY YOUR HEALTH AND HUNGER

You are what you eat. Unfortunately, it's too easy to skip regular meals when you're busy taking care of your family. But you must have glucose to fuel your brain, fatty acids and proteins to maintain cell structure, and vitamins and minerals to support cellular metabolism. You've frequently read or heard what constitutes a healthy diet and how important it is. You know, for example, that you need to eat fewer processed and fast foods and more fresh veggies and ripe fruit. But you still have cravings and individual needs that often arise, especially if things get out of control at home.

WHAT YOUR BRAIN NEEDS

Glucose. Your brain works best with a total of twenty-five grams of glucose in the bloodstream, about the amount in a banana. If you skip breakfast, your blood glucose levels will drop and you won't be able to concentrate after 11:00. You also want to avoid the blood glucose spike caused by eating a candy bar on an empty stomach, because an elevated glucose level also reduces your ability to concentrate. It activates the stress response system, elevates cortisol (a.k.a. the stress hormone), and decreases your performance on cognitive tasks.

Your brain needs a *constant supply of glucose* rather than big spikes from too much sugar. Carbohydrates in your diet provide a *continuous source of glucose throughout the day*, giving a steady supply of energy to the brain.

Fatty acids. *Your brain consists of 60 percent fat.* Fat consists of long-chain polyunsaturated molecules that contribute to the white matter in the brain, which *speeds up information flow.* White matter also repairs cell membranes and manufactures the hormones that regulate heart rate, blood pressure, blood clotting, and immune functioning. These fats are not created by the body. We can only get them from our diet, so they're called *essential fatty acids.* Flaxseed oil has the highest omega-3 and omega-6 content of any nonmeat source. Other dietary sources include other seeds, oily fish, and some dark leafy green vegetables, such as kale, spinach, and mustard greens.

Proteins. Proteins, and the amino acids from which they are built, are essential for maintaining the structure of the brain. We must have the *right amount of amino acids* in order to create enzymes, which act as catalysts for all our biochemical reactions. Finally, amino acids are key components of neurotransmitters, which are vital for communication in the brain.

With the standard American diet, there's no need to worry much about getting enough protein. But Jason, who has been vegetarian most of his life, needs to keep an eye on his protein consumption. When he used the standard formula to figure out how many grams of protein he should eat every day—0.4 times his body weight in pounds—the numbers said that he was getting enough. But he was feeling physically tired and his nails were brittle, both signs of protein deficiency. He decided to add a smoothie made with whey powder as an after-work snack. If you're not vegan, dairy and eggs are good sources of protein; fresh organic tofu, beans, nuts, seeds, and whole grains also provide essential amino acids.

Key vitamins and minerals. Many children and adults are low in two key vitamins—vitamin D_3 and vitamin B_{12}. Vitamin D is a fat-soluble vitamin that helps us absorb calcium and phosphate, two minerals that are essential for bone formation. Vitamin D is vital for cell growth, cell proliferation, cell differentiation, neuromuscular and immune functioning, and the reduction of inflammation. It is so critical to the health of our cells that our body makes its own vitamin D when our skin is exposed to the sun. It's the *sunshine* vitamin. In the summer, if you're fair skinned and spend about ten minutes in the midday sun, your body will produce more than enough of this vitamin. But in the winter, north of Atlanta the sun is so low in the sky that its UVB rays don't penetrate the atmosphere, so you need to take a supplement. The government recommendation is 200 IU (international units) per day, but many nutritional experts recommend up to 2,000 IU per day.

Vitamin B_{12} is another vitamin critical for our brain and body health (red blood cell formation, absorption of nutrients from food, neurological functioning, and DNA synthesis). Vitamin B_{12} is involved in the production of almost one hundred different biochemicals in our body, including DNA, RNA, hormones, proteins, and lipids. It's very rare in plant foods, so if you're vegetarian, be sure to take a supplement; 500–1,000 mcg is recommended.

A fascinating and important area of research that links the ancient findings of Ayurveda with modern science has to do with the importance of the bacteria in our digestive system. The types and the amount of bacteria in our gut can have marked effects on both our brain and our immune system. The community of microorganisms in our gut is called the *microbiome* and consists of about one hundred trillion microbial cells. We have ten times the number of microorganisms in our gut than the total number of cells in our entire body. The microbiome sends signals directly to the brain through the nervous system. It also affects immune functioning, which, in turn, affects the development of our brain. What we eat can change the composition of the microbiome and determine its influence on other parts of our body. This is particularly interesting since one of the main tenets of Ayurveda is that food is medicine and that *good health begins with good digestion.*

RECOMMENDATIONS FROM AYURVEDA

Ayurveda has specific recommendations for diet for each brain/body type, which we have summarized in appendix 1. There you will also find a simple list of suggestions to help improve digestion for all types.

CHAPTER 4

THE THIRD TOOL OF DHARMA PARENTING:

Attention and Appreciation

Tom and Laura adore their brand-new daughter Kim, but already they're getting far more parenting advice than they want: "Don't pick her up—she's just crying to get your attention. You'll spoil her!" "Why are you talking to her? She can't understand you yet." Luckily for baby Kim, they manage to ignore it.

They understand that crying is the only way a newborn can tell them she's uncomfortable, so when Kim cries they try to figure out what she needs. Tom and Laura talk to Kim constantly, explaining what's going on and why they are doing things. They know that hearing Mom and Dad speak not only soothes and calms Kim, but also stimulates the brain development needed for speech.

When Kim is about five months old, Tom is watching as Laura gets her dressed. She holds up two pairs of little corduroy overalls: "Which pair do you want to wear today, the blue one or the yellow one?" Kim looks at her mom, waves her hands around, and accidentally touches the blue overalls. "Great, you want the blue ones. Let's put them on."

Tom is almost rolling on the floor laughing. "She doesn't know what's going on!"

"Of course not," Laura replies, "but at some point she'll figure out that she gets to wear whichever pair she grabs. I want her to know at the earliest possible age that she gets to make choices and that we pay attention to her. I want her to know that we appreciate her as a human being with valid needs and preferences."

And so it goes. When baby brother Mike is born five years later, they consult Kim about his name, what color blankets to buy for him, where to put his crib. When Mike is five months old, Kim is the one holding up his overalls so he can "choose" what to wear. And as Mike grows up, Tom and Laura carefully explain to Kim what he can do at his age, how much he understands, and how she can help him learn. They are careful to give their full attention to Kim and Mike whenever possible. For example, when they're waiting at the dentist they read books together—the whole family can recite Green Eggs and Ham from memory.

As the kids get older, Tom and Laura include them in as many decisions as possible, from what kind of pizza to make on Friday night to where they should go for vacation. Everyone's suggestions, no matter how wacky, receive attention and consideration. They also make sure that both children understand the basic prin-

ciples of brain/body types. Kim knows (for example) that Mike's not running out the door to get away from her— his Vata won't let him be still, and Mike knows that his big sister isn't being slow in order to make him mad— it's just her Kapha nature. Understanding brain/body types makes them more considerate of each other, and also helps them understand their friends better. Because the whole family shares household tasks—cooking and gardening and budget planning—Mike and Kim naturally get good attention from their parents and feel that their help is valuable and appreciated.

By middle school, both kids have started helping with vacation planning: computing mileage, comparing hotels, and keeping track of the budget. In high school they start to cook some of the weekend meals, in return for their parents doing kitchen cleanup. When Kim wants to be homeschooled during her junior and senior years, Laura and Tom listen to and appreciate her reasons, and then massively rearrange their work responsibilities to accommodate her. When Mike wants to drive with two friends to a weekend music festival, they discuss it carefully, and Tom insists that they take along a parent for safety. The boys are reluctant, but it turns out fine; Tom doesn't interfere with their fun, and comes in very handy when the car breaks down on the way home. At high school parent meetings, Laura and Tom are completely silent, while other parents are complaining about their teens' lack of responsibility and antisocial behavior. In contrast, Laura and Tom feel their family is made up of friends who appreciate and enjoy each other, and who work together so that everyone is happy and growing.

This story illustrates two of the most important aspects of parenting: *attention and appreciation*. It's important that you reinforce your children's positive emotions and behavior, especially when you're doing things with them, because attention without appreciation is negative attention. Negative attention is critical and constraining: "Stop doing that! You're just making a mess." "Why are you trying that? Can't you see it won't work?" "Why can't you get better grades? You're just lazy." Comments like these *hurt*. They wipe out self-esteem and inhibit or smother creativity and curiosity. And it's interesting that the result of negative attention to your child's faults and mistakes is often the direct opposite of what you're trying to achieve. Tell your kids they're getting bad grades because they're lazy, and it will become true. Instead, appreciate their efforts by letting them know that you understand how hard school is for them. Give them attention by helping them figure out their homework and encouraging them. This will help motivate them. It may require months of appreciation and gigabytes of attention, but it *will* eventually make a difference.

Athletes understand the power of positive rather than negative attention: When they visualize their performances, they're careful not to visualize a possible mistake or failure. They know that if they do, they may repeat the mistakes in competition, and even make more. In the same way, if we constantly remind our children of their failures and shortcomings, we are belittling their abilities, undermining their efforts, and destroying their self-confidence. If we keep telling them that they're not good enough and will never accomplish anything, they may very well prove us correct. On the other hand, if we want to develop our children's strengths, we must give them positive attention and appreciation. When we focus on their talents and successes, we improve our children's self-esteem and confidence, which naturally improves their performance.

Children do not need *objects; they need your focused and loving attention.* When your child, *at any age,* comes up to you and asks for help, try to immediately stop what you are doing and *listen.* If you can't take time to talk through the whole issue at that very minute, that's okay. *It's most important to respond right away so your child knows that his needs are significant to you, and that he is your first priority.*

NOTE FROM MOM

A CHILDREN'S CARTOON AS A TOOL TO CREATE GREATER SELF-AWARENESS

The vivid and emotionally accessible movie *Inside Out* illustrates the progression of a child's changing consciousness and growing awareness. Immediately after watching this movie, our eight- and nine-year-old grandkids began taking enormous delight in identifying their own *and each other's* changing feelings of joy, sadness, anger, fear, and disgust, and comparing them to the animated characters who represent the emotions of the main character of the film, a little girl called Riley.

By turning emotions into concrete characters, *Inside Out* gives children everywhere a unique window into their own feelings. When we ask our kids, "How are you feeling?" or "Are you feeling okay?" we're asking them to take a look inside themselves and to identify and recognize *how they are really feeling.* We can then help them figure out what's *causing* their feelings. And later we might help them think about what they can do to feel better, to become more balanced and "in tune" with themselves.

In this book we discuss many different ways to cultivate your child's self-awareness. It can be as simple as noticing when certain scenes in a movie or a TV show are making them anxious or fearful. It may be of even greater value to help your son or daughter *notice* what kinds of people and experiences make them feel positive, confident, and hopeful!

There isn't a movie about brain/body types (yet), but in *Inside Out* the Anger character is an excellent representation of an out-of-balance Pitta type, while the Fear character is a good representation of a nervous, out-of-balance Vata type. Unfortunately, there's no character in the movie who represents an out-of-balance Kapha. The Joy and Sadness characters, however, embody emotions felt by all of the brain/body types when they're in or out of balance.

It's interesting that the resolution of Riley's personal crises occurs when she's able to allow herself to *feel* again, and the feeling part of herself with whom she is able to identify at that moment is Sadness. It's the girl's admission of her sadness, which allows her to open up to her parents' love and to her other feelings, so that *all of her emotions can again be in balance.*

Once our children become aware of and understand their own brain/body types, with their particular emotional and physical strengths and weaknesses, we can help them *figure out how to help themselves rebalance and how to restore* their brains and bodies to a more optimal and resilient state—a balanced state in which we may be surprised to find how often Joy is present.

THE IMPORTANCE OF ATTENTION

In 1999 researchers began to study the mental development of children in Romanian orphanages. From infancy, these children were fed and kept warm, but the orphanages were grossly understaffed, and the staff poorly trained. Although the children's physical needs were met (minimally in most cases), they were not nurtured in any way. They weren't held, they weren't talked to, and they weren't taught anything. The study followed the children for twelve years and revealed the cruel and disastrous effects that this lack of attention had on child development. As infants, these children would rock back and forth like caged animals. As toddlers, they would not make eye contact or interact with others, since no one had responded to them in the past. As they grew older, they continued to be withdrawn and avoid interactions. They had severely reduced developmental intelligence scores and were both inattentive and hyperactive. These limitations continued throughout the first twelve years of their lives. Another group of children, who were sent to foster homes and received loving attention from their foster parents, began to recover brain and cognitive functioning. And the earlier they were placed in a nurturing environment, the faster and more completely they recovered.

This is just one of many research studies confirming that the positive attention of at least one caregiver can make a huge difference in normal child development. It could be the mother, father, grandparent—any caregiver in close daily contact with the child. The critical point is that the child spends significant time interacting with that person. Social scientists call this relationship an "attachment relationship." Having at least one healthy attachment relationship creates the emotional support that enables a child to develop. It provides the essential experiences that teach a child how to form healthy relationships with others, find emotional fulfillment, and respond to life's challenges.

Children develop a hierarchy of relationships—primarily with their mother, secondarily with their father, and then with grandparents or other caregivers. Usually the mother-child relationship is the most important in the child's life, but the order is based on *how the main caregiver responds* to the child. If the father or the grandmother, for example, is the one taking care of the child, the primary relationship will naturally be with him.

THE PARENT-CHILD ATTACHMENT RELATIONSHIP

It's important for you to know that it is mostly *your relationship* with your son or daughter that makes him feel secure and protected. This relationship goes much deeper than just physical care, such as feeding and putting the child to sleep. It is about *the quality of your attention.* Your loving attention creates a haven of safety and comfort from which your child can explore his environment. Your positive attention builds this relationship and is *the single most important factor determining your child's emotional stability, cognitive and language development, and sense of self-worth, as well as his capacity for dealing with stress and adversity.* Simply put, *positive attention is a big deal.*

Your response to your baby when he is frightened, ill, or emotionally hurt is a primary element in your relationship. Beginning at around six months of age, infants can anticipate your response to their distress, and shape their own behavior accordingly. If, for instance, you consistently respond to your child's distress promptly and lovingly by holding the baby close and reassuring him, your child will learn to more freely express emotions. The child will also seek you out when frightened and remain with you until he feels safe again. On the other hand, if you respond by ignoring or ridiculing your child's distress, or by becoming annoyed, he will develop quite a different pattern of behavior—avoiding you when distressed and hiding negative emotions.

It's remarkable how deeply children internalize the quality of our attention. And neuroscience explains why: *Each experience is imprinted in the brain in physical form* as neuronal pathways. If a child cries and doesn't receive attention, this triggers the amygdala, which acts like the brain's fire alarm, signaling that something is wrong. The amygdala then sets off the fight-or-flight response, and *part of this response is to be wary and fearful of others*. If this happens to the child repeatedly, it strengthens the brain circuits that support distrust, a lack of desire to interact with others, and a belief that the world is an unwelcoming and even dangerous place.

The latest research shows that our experiences even change our DNA. We're familiar with DNA as the molecules containing bits of information that determine *everything* from the color of our eyes to the size of our feet. But our DNA also determines how we respond to stress. Genetic research is now exploring how genes (segments of DNA) can be turned on and off by different types of experiences and stimuli.

Research has clearly demonstrated that a negative attachment relationship makes children more vulnerable to stress and less able to control their anger, hostility, and aggression. Such children also have low self-esteem, impaired cognitive development, and poorer academic performance. This may continue throughout their lives: a negative mother-child relationship is the most powerful predictor of addiction and mental instability in adults.

Research also shows—as you may already have guessed—that *a positive attachment relationship has a positive effect on a child's development.* For example, one study of altruism in toddlers showed that they were more likely to help an adult—by handing them something they'd dropped—if someone had played with them just before. Another study showed that toddlers who felt more secure were also more likely to help.

Should you let your child cry? Babies can't talk yet, so crying is their only way to communicate with you. They're not crying in order to manipulate you, as some have believed in the past; rather, they are *in distress* and crying out for help. Any concern about "spoiling" or creating dependency is completely unfounded and illogical. How can you spoil a baby by helping it when it needs help? Infants cannot change their own diapers or feed themselves. And how will they learn to soothe themselves if they don't know what it feels like to be soothed? Research shows that it's much better to pick up babies promptly when they start crying. It also shows that if you do this consistently during the first six months of life, then by the time the child is a year old he will naturally:

- Cry less
- Learn how to "self-soothe" and to respond more quickly to soothing
- Form a positive parent-child relationship

This principle doesn't end when children start talking—or when they start school, or even when they start driving or go

off to college. At every age, if your child asks for help, stop
and give him your attention and help. Your kids might not
walk up to you and say, "I really need your help on this." It
may be more of a silent cry for help. You might notice that
they're not their usual bouncy little selves, or not doing so well
in school, or that they've become sullen and irritable. Be careful not to swoop in and fix their problems for them, but
rather, provide support so they can figure out how to solve the
problems themselves, or, if necessary, with your help. Children
won't learn how to approach a problem by sitting around be-
wildered; kids learn by finding solutions, first with your help
and, gradually, by themselves.

HOW A PARENT'S BRAIN CHANGES

The parent-child relationship enlivens a specific circuit in the
parent's brain that is actually called the "parental caregiving
neural network." This very important network includes brain
centers that contribute to emotional stability and decision
making. Enlivening these centers *transforms our thinking* from
that of a self-oriented person to that of a family-centered person. And this shift enhances our ability to "hear" and respond
to the needs of our children.

Parenting stimulates the functioning of two neural networks: one processes emotions such as vigilance and motivation, and the other is involved in social understanding and
empathy. An interesting study measured these networks in
both mothers and fathers. In general, the emotional processing network was more active in mothers' brains, while the
social understanding network was more active in father's
brains. But fathers who were primary caregivers showed brain

functioning more like that of the mothers, and these fathers were also more responsive to their infants. So, *yes, parenting does change the brain.*

MIRROR NEURONS:
CHILDREN DO WHAT YOU DO, NOT WHAT YOU SAY

The special brain cells called "mirror neurons," which we mentioned earlier, are why *children largely learn by imitation.* Twenty-five years ago, researchers found neurons that fire when an individual either performs or observes an action. That's right, the *same* neurons fire whether the person is actually doing something themselves or just watching someone else do it.

This is how young children learn. The frontal lobes of their brains are not yet developed, so they lack the brain circuits needed to logically plan a sequence of actions. Instead, they learn by the more mechanical activation of these mirror neurons. It's a simple mimicking process: monkey see, monkey do.

But mirror neurons go beyond mimicking physical movements. They may be involved in a wide range of functions, including understanding goals and intentions, learning ability, social communication and empathy, language, and self-awareness. For example, young children learn how to carry on a conversation by imitating adults: first one person talks, and then that person listens while the other talks. Have you ever watched preschoolers playing make-believe? They appear to be having a conversation, but their answers are often completely unrelated to what their friends have just said. It seems completely random (and quite entertaining, but try not to laugh out loud). As they grow older, these conversations begin to make more sense.

INSIGHTS ON ATTENTION

Science estimates that there are four hundred billion bits of information activating our senses at any one time; however, we take in only two thousand bits. It is our *attention* that determines which of those four hundred gigabits we perceive. There's a video on YouTube that demonstrates this: Six people are throwing two basketballs around, and in the middle of this activity someone comes in dressed in a gorilla suit. The "gorilla" stands in the center of the group, thumps his chest, and walks out. If you tell people who are watching the video that it's very important for them to count exactly how many times the two basketballs are caught during the video, half of those people will entirely miss the gorilla. Yes, they will. *They literally do not see it.* Counting the basketball tosses takes up all of the two thousand bits they can process, so nothing else makes any impression at all. In the same way, our *attention* highlights certain things in our environment and eliminates others—all the time, every day.

Another insight on attention comes from Maharishi Mahesh Yogi, the founder of the TM technique. He defined attention as the flow of consciousness, or awareness, which moves from one part of an experience to another. And just as sunlight changes the appearance of what it falls upon, so the quality of our consciousness "colors" our experience. This underscores the importance of the second tool of Dharma Parenting, *Heal Yourself,* and how it affects the quality of your attention and appreciation. When we are happy and patient, we enjoy our child's brilliance, and our child basks in the positive quality of our attention. This is why our third tool, *attention and appreciation*, is so important. We can strengthen our child's positive qualities simply by putting our attention on them and appreciating what they do.

In 1963, Maharishi commented,

> *If a mother is very loving to her child and has given her great love to him, and he has made her very happy, the child is saturated with great joy. If the mother asks the child to run an errand for her, the will of the mother becomes an added wave of joy for the child. He jumps up and does what he is asked in a very playful and joyful mood. But if the mother has beaten the child, making him cry, and then orders him to do the errand, her order becomes an additional wave of misery to the child. He will do the action, but under great pressure, and thus the whole thing becomes a burdensome and tedious task for him.* (Science of Being, *176*)

Maharishi often used the expression "Mother is at home" to refer to the deep feeling of complete comfort, confidence, and safety that children naturally feel around their mother. Ideally, we want to extend this feeling so the child feels the same level of self-confidence when Mom is miles away. This involves trust and inner stability, both of which develop in small steps over time.

Help to bring your child's attention to the most positive parts of any experience. Ask your child what he is seeing, feeling, and thinking. Remember that *every experience your child has is changing his brain.*

ATTENTION AND YOUR CHILD'S BRAIN/BODY TYPE

> *It's nine thirty on a Saturday morning and eight-year-old Chris is still in bed.*
>
> *His mom, Jenny, shouts up the stairs, "Time to get up, Chris. You've got things to do."*
>
> *Fifteen minutes later, she walks into his room. "Wake up, sleepyhead! The day's awasting."*
>
> *Chris stirs slowly, then sits up suddenly and says, "I'm coming up from the bottom of the ocean to attack you." Giving his mom a goofy attacking-monster face, he grins sleepily.*
>
> *Jenny has to strain not to laugh. Chris is so lovable, but he's also a little lazy. "Sweetie, you've got homework to do and chores piled to the ceiling."*
>
> *"You don't have to crack the whip, Mom. I'm moving, see?" Slowly, he slides out of bed and into a heap on the floor, from which he looks up at her and cackles.*
>
> *"How about pancakes for breakfast?" he asks.*
>
> *Jenny snorts, but she's smiling as she leaves the room. Gotta love him, she thinks, but her smile morphs into worry lines. Is he ever going to accomplish anything in life? He seems so unmotivated. All he wants to do is read, play video games, and eat. And at eight, he's already overweight.*

Chris has a naturally calm nature and enjoys his daily routine. Even tempered and easy to get along with, he is a typical Kapha. Chris's style of learning is very different from his brother's and sister's. He takes in information slowly, but once he understands thoroughly, he tends not to forget. His daily routine is also different. He has no problem falling asleep, but he does have a hard time getting up in the morning, and it usually takes a lot of nagging, sometimes even threats, to get him going.

As Jenny began to learn more about the Kapha brain/body type, she started to change Chris's routine. First of all, in addition to the occasional outdoor activities he engaged in with his friends, she initiated a daily bike ride that they took together. She also limited his video games to an hour on school days and two hours a day on weekends. And the video time had to be after they'd taken their bike ride and he had walked the dog. She used Chris's love of food to interest him in helping her prepare and cook dinner, and this gave them more opportunity to talk and was a positive experience for both of them. Now Chris is getting better grades, losing weight, and both Chris and Jenny are happier.

Jenny's discovery of her son's Kapha brain/body type allowed her to minimize the activities that would imbalance him and to encourage others that would help him stay in good balance and grow. She used the third Dharma Parenting tool when she changed the quality of her attention to, and appreciation of, her son, instigating activities like bike riding and cooking, which helped Chris and also brought him greater enjoyment and well-being. The purpose of Dharma Parenting is not just to correct what's wrong but also to identify and adopt a pattern of living that supports a happy, healthy, and successful life without strain.

Applying the third Dharma Parenting tool, attention and appreciation, resolves many different challenges at different ages.

FROM BIRTH TO EIGHTEEN MONTHS

Research shows that good attention during this period sets up a strong, stable basis for the child's growth. If children are well cared for between six and eighteen months, then future parenting difficulties or trauma will not have as great an effect on them. If they're not well cared for at this time, the effects show up strongly when they're older, even if they are then in a more nurturing and caring environment.

At this age, one of your major considerations is how to best *organize*—your baby will easily go along with any changes. The main question is: Who do you want to care for your child during these critical months? If both parents are working, or if you're a single parent who must work, you need to find a caregiver who will give your baby the *quality of attention* that you want him to have. And when you manage to find this gem, you then have to consider finances: can you really afford this type of care? Finding a good solution requires a lot of ingenuity and flexibility (luck helps)—but remember, this is only until your child begins preschool.

One strategy might be for you and your partner to adjust your work schedules so that you can handle child care yourselves. Back in chapter 3, Monica and Jason managed to do this: Jason worked weekdays and took care of the girls on weekends; Monica worked weekends and mornings so she could be there when the girls were home on weekdays. In some families, one parent works the early shift and the other works the late shift so that one of them is always home.

Perhaps one of you can work part-time or work from home for half the day and at the office the other half. That way, you will be with your baby for all but twenty hours each week. And because you're only away half the day, you might be able to get some help from your family—could grandparents or an aunt help out? Or maybe a friend or sibling has a baby and you can hire one caregiver for the two children.

You may even want to reach for the stars and have one parent stay at home full-time. This eliminates the worry over finding a caregiver and decreases the stress that results from both of you working full-time while trying to parent. Finances tend to be the biggest challenge in this situation, but it's an investment in your family's future. What can you do to make this a practical option? First, while expenses need to be reduced, there are some built-in savings: no caregiver, no work wardrobe or transportation, fewer restaurant meals. The parent at home might also be able to figure out creative ways to contribute to the budget. In the summer, you might grow flowers or veggies and sell them at the local farmers' market, or you might help out a friend by providing part-time child care. Maybe you have a skill you can use to work a few hours at home with your child nearby: editing, baking, computer programming, or sewing. (Motorcycle repair and metal sculpture probably aren't viable options with a baby around.)

PRESCHOOLERS

How to reach out to your preschooler who isn't used to spending much time with you? Your son or daughter is probably used to a caregiver who defers to him or her, because that's the person's job. Now the situation is different because you have things you must get done. Enlist your kids to help you with everything possible, and sincerely listen to their suggestions. Let them be in charge, or at least ask them, "What do we do next?" Think things through out loud so they can follow your thought process.

If your desires conflict with those of your preschooler—
who wants to go to the playground but the floor needs mopping—explain the situation. Don't just say, "We can't do that
now." Ask your child to help so that the chore gets done faster
(of course, it probably won't). At least it will be clean when
you come home from the playground. But if you promise,
you have to keep your word. If there's obviously no time for
the playground, maybe you can take a quick walk to some
other favorite place. But let your child know ahead of time
that this needs to happen and let the child help think up the
alternatives. Don't make it a clash of wills—*create a cooperative venture.*

When choosing activities, take into account your child's
brain/body type. (Your own too, but in this kind of situation,
your child's is more important.)

Vatas like to move, be creative, and explore new things. Try
exercising or dancing together with your child's favorite song
playing. Craft projects are another option. Run around the
playground together. If you need to keep your child occupied
while you are doing something else, don't expect him to stay
focused for very long. Realize that you're going to be interrupted a lot. So take it easy and let your child show you what
she is doing and receive your praise. Accept your child's interruptions as a compliment, a sign that you're important in your
son's or daughter's life.

Pittas like to learn; they like to be the leader, and to reach
a goal. Cook together—look over recipes together. Let your
kids choose and participate so they get to announce, "Look
what I did!" Or they might help you with a household project,
such as planning and planting the garden. If you need to keep
them occupied, give them a puzzle or something educational
to do.

Kaphas like to help people; they also like to eat, and they're powerful once you get them moving. Physical games are especially good for Kaphas. Throw a ball back and forth or teach them to kick a soccer ball. But with Kaphas, be sure to show them *exactly how to do a new activity, step by step*. A Pitta will rush ahead and try to figure it out, but a Kapha wants to master each step before continuing to the next.

SCHOOLCHILDREN

If your children are old enough to be in school full-time, then the adjustments you need to make are less physical—you don't have to rearrange your work schedule or reconfigure your budget—they are more emotional and mental. It can be a challenge for you to break your long-standing habit of being the authority figure and doing things your way—quickly and correctly.

The first step, as you might suspect, will be to *heal yourself.* If you're impatient or if your keep nagging your children because you worry about everything they do, *work on getting your Vata under control.* Get extra rest; cut down your schedule so you're not always rushing around; stay warm and treat yourself to a few comfort foods. If you're irritable or perpetually angry, ordering your children around to make sure they do things right, *cool down your Pitta.* Avoid foods that are hot and spicy; get enough exercise, but stay out of the sun and be sure to drink enough cool water; keep the AC on at home and in the car. If you're grouchy or feel that it's too much trouble to reach out to your children, *it's time to get your Kapha moving.* Hot and spicy foods are good for Kaphas, and so is vigorous exercise.

Fundamentally changing the way you interact with your child is going to require great inner resources. To boost those resources, we strongly recommend Transcendental Meditation to help you have more energy, think more clearly, deal with stress, and maintain your view of the big picture while you're creatively adjusting your parenting style. Your child can also learn TM if he is ten or older. And there's a "walking technique" for children under ten, which will help them be more flexible and less stressed too. If you're both meditating, it will very much support your desire to begin a new way of relating and working with each other.

When you start making changes, take small steps at first. Your child is used to the way you act and has developed behavior in response. The very first thing you can do is to *be less critical of your child*—after all, his brain isn't fully developed yet and your child doesn't have much experience in life but is still trying to do the best he can. Also, *if your brain/body types are different*, which is completely normal, your child's style of functioning will be fundamentally different from yours—he may naturally be faster or slower than you are, or less focused and more emotional, or not very goal oriented.

Once you realize this, it will be easier for you to cut down (and eventually eliminate) any and all harsh negative comments. Instead of saying, "Your room is always such a mess— if you don't clean it right now, you can't go to Little League practice," you might say, "Looks to me like your room needs cleaning. Are you going to be able to get it straightened up before practice?" You can also offer to help. A fourth grader may not even know exactly what you *mean* when you say, "Clean your room." You need to show him the steps: pick everything up off the floor, put the dirty clothes in the laundry basket, straighten the top of the desk and dresser, and sweep the floor.

At the dinner table, if you ask, "How was school today?"

you're likely to get a grunted "Fine" before your kids shovel in their mashed potatoes and excuse themselves from the table. Try asking questions that can't be answered with one syllable: "What was the best thing that happened in school today?" Your children might be a little gruff because they weren't expecting a real conversation, but after a few tries they'll get used to it—and if you listen and are sincerely interested, they may start waiting for you to ask so they can tell you all about it. If you're sure they're doing well in a particular subject or activity, ask about that—but you don't want to start off asking, "How was math today?" if they're really struggling. Later on, when they're used to sharing the events of their day with you, they'll probably be glad to tell you their miseries and maybe even accept some advice.

Make time in your schedule to go to their games or listen to the new piece they're learning on the piano. Don't overdo the praise—your kids will know immediately if you're laying it on too thick, and do commiserate with their failures. They'll be relieved to hear you say, "You almost made that tough catch—it's amazing how close you came," instead of, "Why didn't you catch that? You let down the whole team."

When your kids get used to having you as part of their activities, you can start asking them to be part of yours. Need to rake the lawn? Ask them for help, then make big leaf piles for them to jump in . . . and rake again. Be creative and have fun! If you're enjoying each other at dinnertime, extend the camaraderie by asking them to help bring the dishes to the kitchen. The older ones can take on responsibilities of their own, as long as you help them learn exactly what to do and make sure that they know how much you appreciate their help and how important it is. It's especially nice if the jobs they do can free you up so you can spend more fun time together.

ADOLESCENTS AND TEENS

Forming more positive relationships with older children can be a huge challenge. They've had years to develop self-defense mechanisms to protect themselves from your criticism. They're also going through tremendous brain and hormonal changes, so they hardly know who they are from day to day. You cannot expect them to be as responsive as a younger child would be.

Even so, your approach should be the same as with younger schoolchildren: Start by breaking your habit of criticism and scorn, and then initiate easy, quiet conversations and listen sincerely. Show genuine interest and offer encouragement in their activities and accomplishments. Find interesting projects or chores that might appeal to your son and daughter, and which you can accomplish together.

IT WILL TAKE TIME . . .

If you've been very negative with your children throughout their lives, the process can be slow going, and they may rebuff you over and over again. Pick the best time, and sit down together so that you can acknowledge that you've been treating them badly, and tell them that you'd like to change. If they seem at all willing, you could ask them where you should start. Again, it can take time for them to trust your sincerity. Keep trying. But if the relationship is really dysfunctional, do not hesitate to consult a professional. (If you don't know a friend who's had success with a family counselor or therapist, your doctor or high school counselor may be able to recommend another professional who could help.)

Attention and appreciation is really a very simple concept:

treat your children as human beings *whose needs and desires are as important and valid as your own.* If you take the time to pay attention, you may find that their growth and development are fascinating and naturally capture your attention. Understanding that because of their age and different brain/body types they have different abilities from yours will help you to appreciate that they're doing the best they can and are growing up to become good people.

NOTE FROM MOM

IT'S MORE IMPORTANT TO BE KIND THAN TO BE RIGHT

After a family discussion about respect, our seven-year-old remarked, "Courtesy is the ribbon on kindness." A typically quirky, poetic thing for this kid to say, which got me thinking that an act of kindness is based on "considering," or thinking about, the feelings or condition of another. And one *big* life lesson in getting along with those we care about is that *it's often more important to be kind than to be right.*

Courtesy is less than kindness but more than being polite. Most of us are so intimate and relaxed with our kids and spouses that it's easy to overlook the value of courtesy, but speaking and behaving with courtesy *communicates and cultures respect, as well as our wish for our loved ones to thrive and bloom!* From toddler to grown-up— and for however many years *a marriage* may encompass— courtesy is a small investment that produces incalculably valuable returns.

Unless your child is running into traffic or in some other immediately critical situation, *within the family, being considerate of feelings really is more important than being right.* We always want to protect the tender feelings of our children, which can be hurt, dulled, or damaged (especially Vatas) by being spoken to harshly or with negativity. This lesson is perhaps most important for Pittas of every age, since it's the nature of Pittas to be strongly attached to being right. Kaphas may be either too kind or too remote to argue—unless they're badly out of balance and the subject directly concerns them, in which case they will probably dig in their heels and become stubborn rather than dominating.

When kids speak and behave thoughtfully, caringly, and politely—when they're *genuinely courteous*—we know that they're both capable of, and interested in, being kind.

CHAPTER 5

THE FOURTH TOOL OF DHARMA PARENTING:

Routines to Improve Family Dynamics

The day begins and Joe, a true Pitta, wakes up just before the alarm goes off. "Your turn to get the kids up," he says to his wife, Mary, going into the bathroom to shower and shave.

Mary rolls out of bed and taps on thirteen-year-old Josie's door. Josie is a Pitta, like her dad, and calls out, "I'm already up, Mom."

Their eight-year-old son, Mario, is Kapha, so he's a little harder to rouse, but he eventually gives his mom a thumbs-up, and she moves on to four-year-old James's door. Instantly awake, James is ready to get up and go—exactly what we'd expect from a Vata. Mary gets him started dressing in the clothes they'd laid out together the night before, and ten minutes later, the entire family is heading for the kitchen.

Josie has emptied the dishwasher and is making toast. Mario brings the milk to the table, which was

set the night before. During breakfast, the family dis-
cuss the upcoming day, encouraging Mary, who will
be giving a presentation to new clients, and sympa-
thizing with Mario, who has a math test. After
breakfast, Joe drives off with James, to drop him at
preschool before going to work, and Mary takes the
older kids to school on the way to her office. Whew!!
It's a good thing that each member of the family is
familiar with his daily routine.

Routines provide a measured pace to *structure* the flow of family life: a daily routine helps your child know *what to do* and *when to do it.* You have to remember that children really do not and, more important, *cannot* grasp the big picture of how their life is organized. First of all, their brains are not mature enough. Their frontal lobes—the part of the brain that synthesizes all their sensory and thought input so they can understand what's going on—are not yet developed fully. Second, they don't have the depth of experience that adults have, so they don't understand how one action leads to the next, in sequence and properly timed. This is the value of a familiar routine for your kids. They can't yet figure out that if they go to bed now, they'll get enough sleep to feel rested when they wake up tomorrow morning. It's much simpler for them to know that after dinner they help with cleanup, then take a bath, brush their teeth, get into bed, and Mom or Dad will read a story.

Initiating routines while your kids are still young is a great help for family dynamics. As they get older, it becomes a little harder to keep them on a regular daily routine. Their schedules get more complex: there's play practice and a basketball tournament and movies with friends. Some nights they go to bed late, and this can affect their routine for days.

As their frontal lobes start to develop, they will naturally want to exercise a more abstract thinking style by considering possibilities and contingencies for how their day may unfold: "Sure, Mom, I'll rake the leaves, but not this morning. I have more energy in the afternoons, you know." This is a delicate time; you don't want to quash their growing independence, but will they really rake those leaves or will they take off with their friends? You may want to relax the usual schedule of Saturday morning chores, yet still give them a deadline, preferably a logical one. "Okay, but a couple friends are coming over at two o'clock, and I'd like the yard to look nice by then." Or offer an incentive: "Do you need a ride somewhere? If you finish by one thirty, I'd have time to give you a drive before my friends arrive."

INDIVIDUAL ROUTINES

There are two types of routines, individual and family. Individual routines are tailored to each person's brain/body type and abilities.

Vata brain/body types, for example, prefer change and variations in life, and will have a harder time following any set daily routine. Vatas, however, actually need routine more than any of the other types because they tend to be so much more spontaneous and less focused. Routines give their natural restlessness (and their creativity) a stable base. When you begin a new routine with your Vata child, it's good to keep a close watch so that he doesn't lose focus and wander off.

Pitta brain/body types generally enjoy routines and order, and when they're in balance they have no problem sticking with set routines—unless, of course, their always-active intel-

lect starts figuring out better alternatives. If their Pitta becomes aggravated, however, they may become rebellious and
resistant to authority of any kind. When you start a new routine with a Pitta child, make sure that they participate in figuring out the details, and be prepared for them to make
adjustments to perfect it.

Kapha brain/body types also enjoy routine—in fact, they
may enjoy it too much. They can become fixated on their
daily schedule and need greater stimulation and new adventures. Introducing Kaphas to a new routine can be quite a
challenge. Kapha kids need plenty of advance notice for any
change. Once you've decided on a new routine together, you'll
have to judge whether your Kapha is eager to start or you
should give him a couple days to get used to the idea. Then
remind your child that the change is about to happen:
"Tomorrow morning, remember, I'm going to wake you up
fifteen minutes earlier so you have more time to eat a good
breakfast. Now, what should we have for breakfast?" Expect
that you'll have to persevere patiently until the new routine is
established. Getting a Kapha to change is like moving a
mountain, but once the mountain has moved, you're all set.

EXERCISE ROUTINES

Exercise is one of the engines that drive optimal growth and
development. Exercise strengthens the body and maintains
cardiovascular health.

If you're very lucky, your kids' routine can include a safe
walk or bike ride to school. Not only does this give them regular exercise in the fresh air, it also serves as "downtime," a
chance to think about their day and decompress. If the walk
to school is too long, see whether you can drop them off part-

way so they'll have a bit of exercise—perhaps on the other side of the football field or playground.

In any case, it's good to put attention on exercise for the whole family. On the weekends, join your kids on family walks or bike rides. Have a picnic in the woods with a nature hike afterward. Or combine exercise with chores that need to be done: gardening, leaf raking, cleaning out the garage or basement. Both excursions and "home" work also allow the family to appreciate one another and learn how to cooperate with others.

When it's too cold for the playground, little ones may enjoy programs like Kindergym, where they learn coordination and play with their friends. When they're old enough, help them find enjoyable physical activities: T-ball, soccer, and ballet are classic choices, but there are lots of fascinating options, like Irish step dance and martial arts. If your kids opt for competitive sports, such as tennis or gymnastics, be very careful not to push them too hard. Not only will they risk injury by trying to go beyond their abilities, but sometimes we, as parents, don't realize how much stress we add to our children's lives when we urge them to win. After a competition, focus your comments on how they performed, not on how well they placed: "Your backhand is really improving," or "Wow, you almost made that back flip on the balance beam—it was amazing to watch."

When you and your child are considering recreational or athletic options, be sure to take their brain/body type into account. Vata children love motion and can develop very refined motor skills. Their grace and agility may lead them to dance and gymnastics. You have to remember that Vatas tend to have limited stamina; they are sprinters rather than marathoners, and may not have the endurance for soccer or basketball. If they choose these sports, monitor their energy level carefully. Volleyball, tennis, or softball/baseball may suit them much better. Vata physiologies are a little more fragile than the other types—their bones are not as sturdy and their muscle mass is lower—so contact sports such as football and martial arts might not be so good for them. If they choose one of these, make sure that their coach is safety conscious and vigilant to prevent injuries. Vatas have a tendency to overdo things, so ensure that your Vata child gets lots of rest and doesn't become overexcited.

Pitta children often think they're indestructible—and they might almost be right. They love competition and have good stamina and strength, so they are often drawn to organized sports. They're so intense that they will naturally push themselves to their limit in any sport or activity, so again, monitor the risks very carefully to avoid injury. And watch out especially for "Pitta perfectionism": If they push themselves too hard, they risk not only physical injury but also mental stress. If they can't meet their own high expectations, they may become overwhelmingly angry at other players and at themselves.

Kapha children can be good athletes because they tend to be very strong, with good endurance, but they're not as energetic and high spirited as Pittas. Physical exercise, however, is critical for Kapha types—it keeps them from becoming lethargic and overweight. Many Kaphas are quite social, so they enjoy the camaraderie of team sports—helping their teammates is a good Kapha motivator. Kaphas have the stamina for soccer and basketball.

The most prominent athletes in popular competitive sports tend to be a combination of both Kapha and Pitta. This type of brain/body type gives a high level of strength, energy, and physical resilience.

AFTER-SCHOOL ROUTINES

After-school routines tend to develop almost by themselves and can change quickly as your child gets older. Regardless of their age, though, children need four things: a nutritious snack, time to decompress from a busy day, time to reconnect with the family, and time for homework.

A nutritious snack. The body has a natural slump in midafternoon, and physiologists talk about "reduced levels of catecholamines," which in English means that your energy and concentration nose-dive. Avoid sugary snacks that perk you up but cause a sugar crash later on. Fruit and high-protein foods provide steady energy and keep you on an even keel.

The stomachs of little ones are much smaller than those of adults, so they need to eat more often. And even when your kids grow taller than you are, their metabolism is fast and they're burning a lot of energy. If you're home with them in midafternoon—whether they are coming home from school, or younger ones staying home—designate a snack time. Plan it as carefully as you would any meal, making sure that it's nutritious, appealing, and appropriate for their brain/body types. Often kids will enjoy helping you make the snack, and as they get older they'll introduce their own creative variations and may even take over completely.

If you can't be home with your children in the afternoons, make sure that their caregiver understands how important the snack is. Give specific instructions, or provide the snack each day.

Older children who stay after school for sports and other activities also need to eat. For example, a fourteen-year-old boy on the football or basketball team needs at least 3,000 calories per day; a girl pursuing an active sport needs about 2,400 calories. By the time sports practice starts, it's been about four hours since lunch, and they're about to burn a lot of energy and need fuel. Sports bars are easy to carry, so is a baggie of roasted sunflower seeds and raisins. Don't forget water! They can carry their favorite water bottle to school and fill it before practice.

NOTE FROM MOM

SNACK STRATEGIES

Vata brain/body types do better with easy-to-digest snacks such as fruit, yogurt, and toasted sunflower seeds. Avoid crisp, dry foods such as potato chips or popcorn, because these aggravate Vata and cause imbalance. Unless it's really hot outside, Vatas do well with warm foods: muffins or cookies right out of the oven, warm drinks such as cocoa and hot cider, a cup of hot soup.

Pitta types have strong digestion; often they'll be roaring hungry by midafternoon and need a hefty snack to quiet the dragon in their stomach. Do not inflame that dragon with hot or spicy foods—cool is much better for Pitta. Yogurt and granola, several muffins and milk, soup with a sandwich: a Pitta's snack can be almost as big as their dinner.

Kaphas have slower digestion and generally don't need much of a snack. Stay away from cold, heavy foods such as yogurt, ice cream, and cheese sandwiches. A crunchy apple, crisp carrot sticks, or a muffin and some fruit juice will often be enough for a Kapha snack.

Time to decompress from a busy day, and time to reconnect with the family. These may happen at the same time or separately. Some kids need time by themselves to relax and unwind; others want to tell you all about everything, and in detail. Be alert to their needs: listen to them if they want to talk, but don't push them to confide in you if they need some time by themselves.

If you realize that you haven't been connecting with your child after school, it's a good idea to start the new habit gradually—you don't want them to feel that you're interrogating them. You can have an informal chat on the drive home from school or at the dinner table. Also, it's important to ask them *specific questions*, not just "How was school?" or "How was your day?" At best, you will receive a one-word answer: "Okay" and maybe a shrug. Instead, ask younger children, "What was the best part of your day? What was the worst?" With older children, ask about the biology test they were studying for or what skills they're working on in basketball practice.

Time for homework. Elementary students typically don't bring much schoolwork home: an arithmetic worksheet, some spelling words to learn, a reading assignment. How closely you supervise them depends on the child. Your focused Pitta may study best in his room, with no interruptions. On the other hand, you might want to keep your Vata at the dining table after snack time to make sure he doesn't go wandering off, literally or figuratively. And you probably want to keep your Kapha student nearby so you can be sure he's working and not just resting or snacking.

In middle and upper school, the pace of homework picks up—and so do the after-school activities. It's a constant tug-of-war between all those wonderful activities, homework, and sleep. Learning takes time and attention; if your kids are trying to cram a chapter of social studies between volleyball and play practice, they're not going to learn effectively. And calculus at midnight isn't going to allow them to absorb much, either then or the next day—because the first thing that shuts down when you're tired is the learning part of your brain. Help your teens keep their schedules under control so they have time to study and time to sleep.

MEDITATION ROUTINE

We recommend including meditation—specifically Transcendental Meditation—as part of your family's daily routine. Forty years of research clearly shows that TM helps enormously in managing stress and anxiety, thinking more clearly, and adapting more quickly and creatively. It's one of the best parenting tools available, and one of the greatest things you can do for your children. Children as young as four can learn a special children's technique, and at age ten they can learn the adult TM technique.

It can be quite a challenge to fit meditation in twice a day. In the morning, getting up earlier is about the only option for most people. We know one high school student who sets her alarm early on school days because she loves the luxury of resting for fifteen minutes after her morning meditation. If the trip to school is long enough, the kids may be able to meditate while you drive. For parents, one option for a quiet, uninterrupted meditation might be to stay later at work and do it there. If you're at home in the afternoon, you could fit it in with your preschooler's nap or quiet time. If the evening isn't too rushed, however, your family can meditate together before dinner; this also works well on weekends.

ELECTRONICS ROUTINES

Electronics can be one of the modern world's trickiest parenting challenges: keeping your children from being *overconnected* with too much phone use, too much web surfing, and having their noses glued to the screen instead of participating in real life. Step one is to lead by example: Are you cemented to your cell phone? How many hours a day do you spend staring at your computer screen? Mirror neurons come into play here: Your kids see you absorbed in the digital world, and their brains automatically set out to copy you. So it's very important for you to strictly follow all the guidelines your family decides on.

Because these guidelines are going to affect every family member who is old enough for a phone or computer, don't hand down pronouncements from on high. Get everyone together, provide a great snack, and hammer out the guidelines. And make it very clear that while these guidelines need to be followed, they're not written in stone. They can be modified to suit each person's needs—but not by wailing, "You can't turn off the Wi-Fi now—I'm skyping with Hayley!" Try out the guidelines for a week and then get together again and decide what needs to be changed and improved.

Consider the following:

- No electronics in bedrooms after bedtime. You might designate a central "charging station" where everyone puts their phones and laptops when they go to bed, whether they need charging or not.
- Turn off the Wi-Fi hub when you go to sleep. You could make an exception when older kids need to work on homework on a school night. But ask them what time they will turn off the computer.

- Your cell phone provider probably has a family plan that allows you to limit phone use: minutes, texting, and data.
- Some families change the Wi-Fi password every weekend; the new password is earned by finishing the weekend chores.

It's important to help your children learn how to entertain themselves without relying on their electronic buddies. Try to start their electronic career as late as possible. Your toddler probably does not need a computer designed especially for that age group. When you buy a minivan or SUV, does each child really need their own DVD player and screen? Electronics are fun to look at and they keep a child occupied with pretty colors and sounds, but what about the other senses? What about playing board games or shuffling a deck of real cards? What about talking to real live people? Instead of movies on a car trip, look out the window, play games, follow your route on the map, and calculate mileage. Prepare for a trip by printing puzzles, mazes, and sudoku from the Internet; these can be tailored to all different ages.

NOTE FROM MOM

HIGHWAY ROUTINE (A.K.A. THE CAR GAME)

This game has kept families occupied on car trips from preschool through college.

It's a cooperative game, not a competition; the object is to rack up as many points as possible by finding things that are on the "points list." Here in the Midwest, we started out with ten points for a water tower and one point for cows (alone or in a herd). You'll want to create your own list, but here are a few things we watch for on our trips. (Over the years, we've developed a list of about twenty "point getters.")

Solar panel: 7 points

Falling-down farm building: 13 points

Horse-drawn Amish vehicle: 50 points

Tractor at work: 6 points

Tractor just sitting: 3 points

Lawn tractor: 2 points

Tractor mailbox: 2 points

(Did I mention we're in the Midwest?)

Everyone reports the points they find to one person, who keeps a running total for the trip. This keeps your Pitta kids happy because they're in charge and they like the challenge of keeping an accurate total. It keeps the Vatas focused so they don't get restless, and it keeps the Kaphas alert. Because it's cooperative, as well as competitive, it pulls the family together as a team.

Adjust the list to suit your location. When we drove through Vermont, we substituted Moose Crossing signs for falling-down farm buildings, and the names of mountains for Amish vehicles.

SLEEP ROUTINES

Bedtime works best if you create a familiar routine that you and your children enjoy. Have a little quiet fun together at the end of the day; all too soon they'll consider themselves old enough to get to bed by themselves. If you've been letting your partner or spouse put the kids to bed, you've been missing out. At least once in a while, take the time and energy to participate in the bedtime routine. Vata children naturally take the longest to settle down and have the hardest time going to sleep, so they need the most attention; Pittas are easier: they'll efficiently get into their pajamas and brush their teeth, but they may take a while to fall asleep because their active minds keep reviewing the fascinations of the day. Kapha kids are no work at all; sometimes it seems that their default state is deep sleep. Get them started earlier because they may slow almost to a standstill by the time they crawl into bed. And have them brush their teeth right after dinner; if they wait until bedtime, they may be too tired to do a good job.

To help their minds settle down for sleep, stop all TV, computer use, and electronic games at least half an hour before bedtime. The light from these screens tricks the brain into thinking it is still day, so the brain signals the body to stay active. If we turn off the electronics, the brain will realize it's getting dark out there and tell the body to start settling down to sleep.

An easy way to accomplish this is by having your child take a bath or shower at least half an hour before bedtime. A warm oil massage before the bath will pacify Vata and help the muscles relax. The warmth of the bathwater also helps the body relax and settle down. (Electronics should, obviously, be left outside the bathroom.)

The next step is getting your child into nightclothes. One father found a good way to get his seven-year-old son to put on his pajamas: "Wrestle those pajamas to the ground! Pin 'em down! Make 'em real tired." His son could then easily put on his pajamas because they were so weak from wrestling with him!

Reading to children is nearly a universal bedtime routine. See what works best for your family. Keith read the entire Adventures of Tintin series to all four of his children, and Fred read the Harry Potter books to his three girls before bed. As they get better at reading, kids who enjoy being read to will naturally want to read the books themselves. Be ready for change, but at the same time keep routines dependable.

If your child has trouble getting to sleep, try Ayurvedic aromatherapy. Gently rubbing the soles of the feet with warm sesame oil or olive oil is also soothing—but make sure the kids are firmly and finally in bed before you do it, or wearing socks, to avoid oily tracks across the floor.

FAMILY ROUTINES

MEALTIME ROUTINE

Mealtime is family time—meals may be the only time that the family can all be together some days. This is when you can share and review your experiences, discuss plans for tomorrow, and talk through any concerns. But keep the conversation congenial and constructive. Besides nourishing your invaluable family bond, mealtime conversation can be a workshop for kids to learn how to communicate in a group.

Think about your typical family dinner conversations: Does everyone join in? Or do the adults dominate, talking to each other, while the children sit quietly eating? Do the kids tend to misbehave at the table and scurry away at the end of the meal? They can't take part in the adult conversation because they don't really understand what you're talking about, so they may be pinching each other because they have nothing else to do, and leaving because they're happier elsewhere.

If you want to make a change, do it gradually. With younger children, you could try a communication routine we call the Good List. Ask your child:

1. What was the best part of your day?
2. What was the medium part?
3. What was the worst part of the day?
4. What do you think you learned today?
5. What are you thankful for today?

The Good List dialogue gives you an opportunity to explore your child's reality. You could also ask, "How did that make you feel?" or comment, "Weren't you lucky that . . ." These simple exchanges allow your child to share their everyday experiences with you, and let you appreciate their growing sense of self.

With everyone's packed schedule, especially as the kids get older and have more after-school activities and sports, it isn't always possible to sit together for a leisurely dinner. A different time of day might work better. We all know that a nutritious breakfast is important; can you all get up a little earlier and eat breakfast together? Set the table the night before, and if you've got at least one early riser in the family, put him on breakfast duty. Or if your kids are older, maybe you have a cup of herbal tea or cocoa (or something cooler in the summer) about half an hour before bedtime. It's a nice way to wind down, talking over your day together and making plans for tomorrow.

Mealtime routines can include preparing for the meal. There are jobs in the kitchen for every age: even the little ones can put place mats and silverware on the table and let the rest of the family know that dinner is ready. As they grow, they can graduate to tossing the salad, filling water glasses, and carrying out the food. Get them interested in cooking while they're young, and they'll repay you many times over. Salad dressing or no-bake cookies are a great way to start—your kids don't have to use the oven, measurements don't have to be exact, and everyone will appreciate their efforts.

Many families begin their meals by saying grace together. When we sit quietly to give thanks, we settle both our minds and our bodies from all the day's activities, and prepare ourselves to enjoy the food. You may already have an appropriate practice, but if not, try experimenting with different styles of expressing gratitude for your food and see if it has a good effect on your family.

NOTE FROM MOM

MIX IT UP A LITTLE

Routines are great tools for keeping family life running along smoothly. The only trouble with routines is that they're so . . . routine.

Every so often, throw the schedule out the window and take off for some family fun. Ditch the Saturday chores—the bathrooms look pretty clean and you can do the laundry tomorrow—in favor of the petting zoo or a jazz festival or the state fair. You don't need to wait for a special event. Create your own: an afternoon of sledding, snowball battles, and hot cocoa, or an overnight campout. The whole family will be energized and refreshed, and the next week's routine won't seem so routine.

After the meal, there's the inevitable cleaning up to do, but it goes quickly and can even be fun if everyone contributes.

When your kids are quite young, they can bring their plates, cups, and silverware into the kitchen in one or two short trips. As they get older, they can clean off the dishes and put them into the dishwasher, and separate the compostable garbage if you've got a compost pile. Kids can wipe off the table, wipe down the counters, and set the table for breakfast. As with any routine that involves the whole family, *group activities transform necessary daily chores into family fun.* Take turns choosing music to play during cleanup. If you have teens who need to start their homework, they might be excused from cleanup in return for some weekend chores such as laundry or yard work.

WEEKEND CHORES

On the weekends, everyone can pitch in with the household upkeep: cleaning, laundry, yard work, and gardening. Let everyone have a specific job that they choose during family meetings. If it's possible, begin as a group, even though each family member may have separate jobs. Motivation may or may not be everything, but it helps. "If we finish cleaning the living room and mopping before eleven thirty, we'll have time to make cookies for lunch." Or "If we can get the garage tidied up by three o'clock, I'll have time to take everyone to the park for Frisbee golf."

This kind of family routine obviously has a practical value: working together helps make the time go more quickly, and team spirit helps you do a better job. Sociologists use the term "social facilitation," which simply means that *when we do things with others, we do them better.* You've probably noticed that when you're around other people, you tend to be just a little more alert and a little more thorough.

NOTE FROM MOM

BRIBES OR MOTIVATION?

A **bribe** is something you give someone to tempt them to do something they shouldn't do. Example: You bribe your child's teacher to give them an A, or you bribe their coach to let them play in the big game. **Motivation**, on the other hand, is a very useful parenting tool. Up to age twelve, children's brains simply don't work well with abstractions; they can only understand concrete objects, which are here right now, not in some distant future (like next week). For example, avoiding cavities is too abstract to motivate them to brush their teeth; having a clean room doesn't motivate them to keep it tidy. Make the motivating reward concrete and logical: "If you brush your teeth right now, we'll have extra time to read before lights out." Or "Wow! Your room is pretty tidy already. It will hardly take any time at all to clean it, and then you can ask Chris over to play." Try not to use food as a motivator. If your child gets food imprinted as a reward, then as they get older they may use food to reward themselves, causing weight problems. Much better to use an activity to motivate: if we finish this quickly, we'll have time for the playground (or Frisbee or a tennis match).

Be careful, of course, not to overdo it, especially as they get older and their brains are functioning more abstractly. You don't want them to demand a reward every time they do something right. But especially with the littler ones, you can help keep them on task by motivating them with a concrete reward. Often the best reward is getting to spend some extra time with you.

When the family works together, it's easier to keep everyone organized and on task, and chores are more fun. Once the kids are old enough for soccer and dance and T-ball, Saturdays are going to be harder to organize. Not only will your kids be gone part of the day, but *you* will be busy driving them around. Take some time near the end of the week—maybe Thursday after dinner—to look ahead at the weekend: Who needs to be driven where, and when? Can they carpool? When will they do their weekend chores? Can they finish the chores on their own, or do they need a parent (or older sibling) to work with them? Thinking through the schedule ahead of time will make the weekend much calmer, and the chores much more likely to get finished with minimum fuss. Try to create room in the schedule for family time too.

SHOPPING ROUTINES

Karen has a long list of errands for the day, and she has to take five-year-old Derek and nine-year-old Courtney with her. She starts off by making sure they eat a snack before they leave; she also has granola bars and water bottles in her bag because she's learned from experience that hungry kids can get cranky on long shopping trips. On the way to the grocery store, they all talk about what they'd like to eat next week, and Karen makes mental changes to her shopping list. Before they get out of the car, she tells them, "If you can help me choose the food and don't create a fuss, we can stop at the library on the way home." The grocery list is long, but Karen keeps both kids occupied helping her find different items (most of which she could find faster by herself).

Next on the list is the mall. "Can we go to the toy store, Mom? Please, please, Mom?" Karen has been hoping for a quick stop but reflects that Derek and Courtney have adjusted their days to accommodate the household shopping, so it seems only fair that she accommodate some of their desires.

"Sure, but first I have a list of things we need to buy. If you help me with that, it will go faster and then we'll have time for the toy store. But we're not going to buy any toys today. It's a looking day, not a buying day." The three of them zoom through Karen's list, then stop to eat the protein bars she brought and drink some water. Outside the toy store, Karen stops and asks Derek, "What kind of day is today?"

Courtney prompts her brother, "Is it a looking day or a buying day?"

Derek knows the answer: "It's a looking day."

"That's right," his mom tells him. "You can pick out two toys you like, and I'll tell people you want them for your birthday, but today we're not going to buy any toys."

The kids chime in, "Because it's a looking day!"

Karen used several strategies to help the long day go smoothly:

- **Snacks:** Children have faster metabolisms and smaller stomachs than you do, so they need to eat more often. Keeping a little attention focused on this can work miracles to save you from in-store tantrums. Karen fed both kids a snack before they left, and they stopped for another snack when they started lagging a bit.
- While they were still in the car—*before* they entered the mall—Karen gave the kids a **simple run-through** of what *was* going to happen and what *wasn't* going

to happen. For example, Karen agreed to go to the toy store but she made it clear that they would just be looking, not buying. This is especially important if you're shopping with young children who have not had a lot of experience in large stores.

- **Motivation:** Another preshopping strategy Karen used was motivation: "If you can help me pick out our groceries for the week and don't create a fuss, then we can stop at the library on the way home." Or you could offer ice cream (or hot cocoa in winter). This creates a win-win situation, since you will all benefit from sitting and recharging after shopping. Be sure to use specific, concrete terms for what you expect from the children: "Be good," or "Be polite," or "Be nice" are much too abstract for kids to understand.

- **Buzz phrases:** Children like buzz phrases because they are easy to understand and easy to remember. For example, Karen repeats, "What kind of day is today? Today is a *looking day*, not a *buying day*." Catchy phrases can be lifesavers on the storm-tossed sea of our daily encounters. They won't always work, but if you repeat them, your child will understand the principles better, and even enjoy them.

- **Participation:** While you're shopping, you make dozens of decisions. This isn't at all interesting to watch, but it is interesting to participate in, so involve your children in the shopping process. Even a toddler sitting in the shopping cart's seat can hold a package of cheese if you tell her, "I need you to take care of this for me. It's for our cheese sandwiches when we get home." Preschoolers can find items for you on the lower shelves, and older kids can read the signs to see whether you need to go down that aisle or not. Whatever their age, try to involve your kids in the process; ask their opinion and respect their answers. "The pineapple is on sale today. How many should we get? Do we want crushed to put on our ice cream, or slices for pineapple upside-down cake?" Helping to make decisions not only keeps kids focused and by your side, so they're more likely to behave well, it's also good practice for making more important decisions as they get older. You are also mentoring them in how to make good choices by taking them through your thought processes as you figure out what to buy.

FAMILY MEETINGS

Every family has many issues that need to be discussed: everything from chore assignments to curfews to vacation plans. Some families can do this informally, just talking things over at mealtimes or during car trips. Others find that they function better in a routine of family meetings. The best way to approach scheduling is to make a fixed time for family meetings, either once a week or once every two weeks, in a place that is both comfortable and orderly, perhaps sitting around the dining room table. You may want to make it part of a fun family night, with games or a movie and snacks after the meeting.

Basic rules for family meetings might include:

- **Regular meetings.** If you have weekly meetings, then no one has to remember what day it's on, which is a real plus. Meetings can last from fifteen minutes to an hour. Some meetings can include brainstorming sessions, when the family generates a list of ideas without any evaluation.

- **Have an agenda that includes topics of interest to everyone.** Post the list on the refrigerator several days ahead so everybody can see the points and add any new topics that are important to them.
- **Everyone must attend.** If the whole family isn't there, it isn't really a family meeting. Of course, there should be some flexibility. But the intention is that the family meets together.
- **All cell phones and other electronic gadgets are turned off.** Kids are tied tightly to their electronics, and it's good for them to experience face-to-face interactions that help develop social skills.
- **Start each meeting with appreciation.** One of the real bonuses of family meetings is that each person has an opportunity to say something good about everyone else, and hear something nice about himself or herself. Keep this part short and sweet, especially in a large family, or it could take up the whole meeting. It may seem silly to start the meetings by having everyone give compliments, but *it helps teach your children to focus on the positive rather than the negative, and to uplift rather than criticize each other. It also encourages family unity and team spirit.*
- **Go through each agenda point.** If a topic is particularly important to one of the children, it's good to begin with that. And each member should have equal time in presenting his opinion. A one-minute egg timer will help keep anyone from talking too much. During the timed period, everyone should listen. This is simple courtesy and teaches respect for others.

- **Review the week.** You can bring up things that may
  not have gone well during the week. But don't spend
  a lot of time on *why* something wasn't done right, or
  who was responsible; instead discuss *how to do it differently in the future.* It's often easier to deal with complicated, difficult issues in the loving atmosphere of a
  family meeting than right at the moment they happen. There's an expression, "Teach away from the moment." This means only deal with the immediate
  pressing issues of any upsetting situation at the time.
  Help your kids *learn from the situation at another time,*
  such as during a family meeting when heads are cool
  and hearts are warm. If you really need to discipline
  someone, it's much better to do this privately. The
  meeting is for deciding guidelines and consequences,
  not for discipline. *Family meetings are the best time to
  discuss what the consequences should be for inappropriate
  behavior.* The idea of family meetings is to *involve the
  kids in the decision-making process.* Children are far
  more willing to obey rules if they help create them.
- **Decisions should be made by consensus.** This is key.
  Families are not dictatorships. They're a group of people living and growing together, and everyone is an
  individual with needs and preferences. By honoring
  each child as a person with valid concerns, the family
  grows stronger. It may take more than one meeting to
  resolve an issue, so don't be pressed to come to quick
  conclusions.
- **End the meeting with something fun.** This could be
  treats or a short game. Or you might morph your
  meeting into a full-fledged family fun night, with a
  movie, games, and snacks.

Brain/Body Types at Your Family Meetings

Family meetings are a great opportunity for kids to learn self-expression, respect for others, decision making, and leadership skills. Brain connections are changing in your child every second, so the dynamics of the family meeting will also change continually. Try to remember that what worked yesterday may not work today or tomorrow, so *be flexible* in your meetings. Some families never have a formal family meeting, while others use them to keep everyone organized. You might switch from formal to informal meetings, depending on your children's ages and circumstances.

During family meetings, be aware of how each of the different brain/body types are likely to interact. Without meaning to, Vata children will tend to speak out of turn and go on too long. This is an opportunity to provide a setting in which they can learn not to interrupt others and to wait their turn while others talk. This is not easy for Vatas, but so necessary. Family meetings are also a chance for all of the children to practice speaking clearly and concisely. Vatas are full of creative ideas, but they need to learn how to communicate them in an effective and courteous manner.

A Pitta child (or parent) will naturally tend to dominate any group. They love to lead, and their Pitta intellect can come up with many solutions to any situation. It's your responsibility to make sure they don't take over the family meetings. This experience will help your Pitta children develop their leadership skills and learn how to work cooperatively with a group.

Kapha children take extra time to get used to any new situation, so they may not contribute much when you first start holding family meetings. Don't push them to be the leader or the secretary. Once they become comfortable and know what's expected of them, they'll often help everyone stick to the agenda and also maintain harmony among the different family members. Watch out, though, because Kaphas can be stubborn and refuse to compromise once they've figured out their position on an issue. Give them time to change—maybe table that issue until next week's meeting.

DAILY ROUTINE WALL CHART

You will want to create a chart for each child, laying out the daily routine, and taking into account the child's age and brain/body type. Let them make it their own by decorating it with stickers and crayons, or other creative touches. The great value of putting routines into a chart is that your child can simply *look* at it in order to know what to do with no worrying about making a mistake, or what's right or wrong. What to do and when to do it are there in black and white, or maybe pink and blue and green.

For young children, the chart could be an arts and crafts project you do together, with pictures from magazines, drawings, and photos, as well as words. You want the chart to *clearly show* each thing that needs to be done in your child's life from morning to bedtime, including: brushing teeth, dressing, breakfast, getting to school, after-school snacks, tidying the room, bathing, getting into pajamas.

Routines require caring, thought, creativity, and flexibility, and they work best when your kids help create them. Once everyone becomes familiar with them, routines provide a framework that allows your children to understand what is going to happen and what is expected from them. Like everything else in the real world, routines have to be reviewed and tweaked periodically to accommodate your children's changing brain connections, their ever-increasing interests and activities, and your own situation. Routines need to grow with your family, and your family will grow on the stable ground of routines.

CHAPTER 6

THE FIFTH TOOL OF DHARMA PARENTING:

Manage Meltdowns and Cultivate Behavior

It's the middle of A gorgeous sunny summer day, and Maryanne glances out the kitchen window to see her nine-year-old son Paul and his buddy, Chris, building a fort in the backyard. All of a sudden, a commotion erupts and she hears Chris complain loudly, "You're not playing it right. I'm the king and you're the knight. You have to do what I say!"

"No, I don't," Paul responds. "Get out of my fort!"

Maryanne rushes outside and puts herself between the two boys. Now what?

Valerie has been in a state of excitement since she received her acceptance letter from college, where she plans to double major in art and dance. So her mom is surprised when the girl rushes into the living room

sobbing, "I can't do it! I can't possibly go to college in the fall!"

Enveloping Valerie in a hug, Mom asks what's wrong.

"I have to choose my freshman seminar topic this week, and whatever class I choose, that professor will be my adviser, so it's really, really important, and all the classes look great, and I was thinking of taking a class that doesn't have anything to do with art—just for fun, to explore something different—but then my adviser won't be in the art department." She turns to her mother and wails, "I don't know what to do!"

Karl has always been the catcher for his Little League team, and his dad is the coach. But because the first baseman had the flu today, Karl had to play first base—not his favorite position, especially on short notice. To top it off, his team lost by one run. His dad helped him feel a little better by praising him in the after-game meeting, for hitting in a run and saving a couple of wild throws.

But they're not at home for ten minutes before Dad hears a roar from the kitchen: "I was saving a bowl of mac 'n' cheese from lunch for my snack and now it's not here. Who ate it?"

Striding across the kitchen, Karl catches sight of the empty bowl in the sink, and throws it on the floor, scattering broken crockery everywhere.

Perhaps the stereotypical meltdown is a Pitta preschooler throwing a tantrum in the middle of a busy store, but meltdowns can happen to any brain/body type, anywhere, and at any age. A meltdown calls for quick, decisive action from you, the parent, so it's essential for you to understand what caused it in the first place.

Remember, the emotional part of our brain develops before the reasoning part (the frontal lobes, the executive control system) that keeps it in check. This means that your child's brain is very easily taken over by feelings of frustration, anger, or anxiety, *and it's not unusual for a child's wish or desire to become so strong that it overrides everything else.* Kids simply cannot control the impulsive, emotional centers of their brain: when their Pitta goes out of balance, they can't control their anger; when their Kapha is out of balance, they can't control their stubbornness or possessiveness; when their Vata is aggravated, they can't control their anxiety or restlessness.

This is a very important concept for parents to grasp: meltdowns are often *triggered* by a problem, but the out-of-control surface behavior you're witnessing is not the *root cause* of the meltdown. A meltdown happens not so much because of a problem or an event itself, but because your child is imbalanced—too tired, too anxious, or too hungry—to use his brain and social skills to deal with the situation. Since you can't solve a problem on the level of the problem, the first thing for you to do is *deal with your child's brain/body imbalance.* Help your child reach a calmer, more balanced, and composed state. The problem might then take care of itself. And if it doesn't, a calm child will certainly be better able to work with you toward a solution. For example, nine-year-old Paul's meltdown was clearly caused by overheating, which aggravated his Pitta. After accurately identifying the problem, his mom sim-

ply said, "It's time for a snack. How about a popsicle?" She
then took the boys into the air-conditioned house, where they
ate their snack and had a good time watching a favorite movie
together. Valerie's case is different. Once she calmed down, she
still had to choose her freshman seminar class, and Valerie and
her parents discussed her choices over several days before she
was able to make a final, balanced decision.

To help you manage meltdowns and modify inappropriate
behavior, Dharma Parenting recommends six steps, *all beginning with the letter C:*

- **Check in** with yourself and with your child.
- **Comfort** your child.
- **Change** your child's brain state.
- **Choices:** Give choices.
- **Consequences:** Enforce consequences.
- **Coach:** You're the coach.

Here's how to calmly use the six C's to get your child back
in balance and smiling again:

1. Check in with yourself and with your child

First of all, check in with yourself. We know that it's not
always easy to do this, but it's essential: When you recognize that you're upset, try to keep your mouth closed and
don't say anything until you're calm. Take a deep breath.
Count to ten. Do whatever you need to do to consciously
slow down and shift gears. Quickly assess the needs of your
own brain/body type: Are you a Vata who's trying to do
too much in too little time, or on too little sleep? Are you
a Pitta who missed lunch? Realizing that your emotional
reaction is tied to your own brain/body imbalance can

help you step back enough so you can deal with the situation more calmly, objectively, and effectively.

NOTE FROM MOM

IF YOU SPEAK WITH ANGER

When we react to our son or daughter with anger, with harsh or severe words, or even with a rough voice, we have the same emotional and physiological effect on our beloved child as a bully or a tyrant. *Our anger acts on our child's brain*, initiating a fight-or-flight response, which either makes the child's behavior worse or freezes the child into terrified submission. This is not the kind of parent any of us wants to be.

Try to appreciate for a moment what our children experience when we lose it. Suddenly the big, all-powerful adult they trust most in the world, the one who's been taking care of them, feeding and nurturing them, sharing special moments, and supporting their every endeavor, *becomes a fiery monster*. Our eyes are now glaring at them with anger and frustration. Our voice, which can be so tender and loving, is now spewing commands and insults. Adult anger is *toxic* to children.

As our kids grow older, yelling at them or spanking them occasionally may seem like effective forms of discipline and punishment. *This is a giant mistake!* And we encourage you to refrain from resorting to such shortsighted responses. Inevitably, they will cause far worse problems in the long run. The logic is irrefutable: *How can we tell our children to stop hurting other kids' feelings, and/or actually hitting them, if we're hurting our kids' feelings and/or hitting them?*

The very first step is always to check in with yourself and find even a little calmness inside. This is within your power as an adult; it's a choice you can make. And when you do speak, speak *quietly* and *slowly*.

After you check in with yourself, the very next thing you want to do is to *check in with your child*. Ask yourself: What is my daughter experiencing that makes her behave this way? What's the *cause* of this behavior? Take into consideration your child's particular brain/body type and specific needs.

Vata brain/body types are extremely curious and want to explore everything; they need to keep that busy, creative Vata brain occupied. If they have to accompany you on a long shopping trip, they can start to feel trapped and bored—they've got to move, do something different, or they can become frustrated and overly emotional. Because Vatas also tend to worry, they can have anxiety attacks that manifest as anger and inevitably tears.

If your child is even partially Pitta, ask yourself if he is hungry or overheated. When Pitta children go out of balance, it's usually because their Pitta element has been aggravated by hunger and/or overheating. In either of these states, the child quickly becomes susceptible to anger, aggressiveness, hitting, and temper tantrums. Ice cream is a fast and virtually guaranteed remedy to quiet internal Pitta fire, or you can give them the protein bar you thoughtfully brought along. If your Pitta is bundled up in a parka and scarf, taking off a couple of layers will help the child cool down.

A meltdown can also be inflamed if your child has recently witnessed a heated argument or watched a violent TV show or movie. The memory of such images and sounds may still be lodged in their mirror neurons, so those brain circuits are primed and ready to be expressed.

Address the reason for the meltdown without a lot of talk: "Here, let's cool you down." "I think we all need to take a break. Where shall we sit to eat our snack?" Sometimes this is enough to soothe and rebalance your child.

2. Comfort your child

Regardless of the cause or the size of the upset— from not wanting to leave a friend's house to getting a D on a calculus test—your child needs to know that you're still supporting him. Let your child know this right away. Maybe give a long bear hug or just a touch on the shoulder. You might say, "It's okay. I'm here for you. We'll figure this out. Everything's going to be okay," or "It's all right—take it easy." At such moments your child doesn't have a stable center, but you can bring steadiness, groundedness, to the situation. Your touch and your voice—even if your child shrugs you off or lashes out at you—will let her know that part of her world is loving and supportive, no matter how badly she may be feeling. Your calmness and comfort provide a calm, solid foundation so your child can calm down and work through their meltdown.

3. Change your child's brain state

Young or old, everyone has two possible types of re-sponses in any situation. Neuroscience calls these the "low-road" and "high-road" responses. The low-road state is our "gut reaction," our reflexive response to any experience. It's immediate because there's no processing involved, just instinct. The low road generates a strong emotional response and can totally take over the brain. In contrast, the high road is our thoughtful response; it's part of our critical thinking and planning processes. But because more neurons are involved, it takes more time to make a high-road decision. These two states combine to create our experience of the world.

When kids are in the middle of a meltdown, their low-road state has taken over. It's even possible that they *can't hear you*, and they definitely cannot reflect upon the situation. Their rational, high-road circuits go offline in the heat of the moment. Children simply cannot change their behavior when overwhelmed by strong emotions, and the high-road brain function is completely overshadowed.

So, before you do anything further, you need to change your child's brain state from low road to high road. The low road leads to your child's stress response, to meltdown. Any child who's in an extreme state of internal agitation, impatience, anger, and distress is completely unable to sit quietly. *Something's got to give.* It may be that you can sometimes find a very simple brain/body–based way to *turn down* your child's low-road emotional centers and *turn on* their high-road thinking centers. Try cooling down an overheated Pitta—unzip the jacket, move the child out of the sun, offer a snack and a cool drink. If your Vata is starting to become fidgety and impatient, find some sort of arts and crafts project, or even a coloring book, to engage their creativity. Or maybe there is a place to run around or an indoor playground at the mall. If your Kapha is growing stubborn or possessive, a little exercise, especially with a buddy, may also help him to move toward a more balanced state. Or a snack—even the promise of one—may cheer the child up and induce more flexibility.

If children feel unsafe or uncomfortable, they will continue to be anxious and irritable, which keeps them on the low road. A noisy or busy environment can also keep them agitated and stuck on the low road. If you can't find a quick solution to help change your child's state, change their location. Move the child to a quieter place, but be sure to do it *calmly*; scolding or yelling is completely counterproductive. If you're fighting a fire, the last thing you want to do is add fuel! If you happen to be in the store, pick up your screaming child and carry him back to the car or some other quiet, safe place and sit peacefully together until the child is able to quiet down. Do not leave your child alone in the car. If you're at home, take your child to his room for a little while to settle down.

Wherever you are, do *not* try to talk until your child's *brain state has changed*. Your child *needs* to settle down. If she tries to speak amidst sobs or screams, tell her kindly, "*This is a time for resting, not for talking.* Talking is for when we're quiet and calm. Right now, I'm going to sit here, and we're not going to talk until you can show me that you're feeling calmer." With older children, once they start to settle down you may be able to remind them of their brain/body state: "Hey, this is quite a Vata anxiety attack you're having. Let's get you calmed down and feeling better. Would you like a cup of tea or cocoa?" Recognizing your own state helped you when you checked in with yourself, and it can also help your child. On the other hand, don't be surprised if it doesn't work—remember that even usually mature teenagers may revert to primitive brain states when they get upset.

Michele Borba's *Big Book of Parenting Solutions* mentions an imaginary device called a Temper Thermometer, which allows children to rate their own anger on a scale of one to ten, where one is as relaxed as sleep and ten is volcanic anger. Once your child starts to calm down, it may help to ask what number the Temper Thermometer is reading now. This process *allows* kids to be more self-aware, and this helps improve their brain state. It might be that you'll find it works better with teens, whose self-reflective circuits are beginning to mature, and with girls, who have more connections between their emotional centers and their thinking brain than boys.

Humor can also help change your child's brain state—and yours too. When you "get" a joke, your brain has a specific response that makes it momentarily more alert and creative. This turns on the high-road response, which is exactly what you're trying to do. For example, Karl's dad might say to him, while they're sweeping up the shards of his missing bowl of mac 'n' cheese, "You know, I've got some really good glue down in my workshop. Do you think Mom would notice if we glued these pieces back together and put the bowl back in the cupboard?" Or Valerie's mom might laugh a little and say, "I'm thinking of Grandma—what would she say if she could see us in tears about having to choose classes at your number one choice of colleges? She'd give us such a hard time, and she'd be so proud of you."

4. Give choices

Once your child has calmed down and more high-road thinking starts to come online again, keep the child on that high road by offering choices. If your child is only partially calmed down, the choices may be quite simple: "Can you finish the shopping without fussing, or should we go home now?" "Do you want to look at the seminar list now or wait until later?" Of course, you have to be realistic in the choices you offer; if you must finish the grocery shopping now, then you can't offer to take your child home first. In such a case, keep the child on the high road by thinking up a couple of realistic choices: "Now that you're feeling better, I really need to do the grocery shopping. Which end of the store shall we start at, the produce or the pasta?"

Another useful tactic is to *divert* them with the choices you offer. Instead of focusing on the trigger that set off the meltdown, *change the subject*: "When does soccer season start? Who's the coach this year?" or "Mom and I've been thinking about summer vacation. How about camping this year?" Changing the subject gives kids something to refocus on and helps to keep the high road active.

Karl's dad used this tool when he walked into the kitchen and found the floor covered with pieces of the broken bowl. On his way to the kitchen, he had checked in with himself and taken a couple of deep breaths to calm himself down. He also checked in with Karl's brain/body state and realized his son's Kapha was way out of balance: First, the boy had to play first base instead of his accustomed catcher position, and Kaphas have trouble with sudden changes. Second, Karl was upset because his team had lost the game. The disappearing macaroni and cheese was the last straw and sent him over the edge. Karl was hungry, and his possessive Kapha nature aggravated the offense: That mac 'n' cheese was *his*. How dare someone else eat it? Dad offered comfort by giving him a quick hug and saying quietly, "Hey, what's going on here? Can I help?"

Karl was desperately upset, and his father knew that calming him down would be a major project, so Dad skipped the step of *calming* him down and gave his son a *choice*: "Look at those sharp pieces on the floor. We've got to get them cleaned up before Salty (Karl's new puppy) comes in and cuts her paws. One of us should shut Salty in the bedroom, and the other can get the broom." This immediately necessary action pulled Karl out of his low-road state, giving him a choice to make, and he decided to go find Salty while Dad got the broom. By the time he made it back to the kitchen, he was starting to be able to think more rationally. Dad gave him another choice: "I'm really hungry too. Shall we make more mac 'n' cheese or split a pizza? It can cook while we clean up."

5. Enforce consequences

Some meltdowns dissolve with few consequences. Your child was out of balance and got upset; you helped him get back on track; now both of you might even feel a little better because you spent some time together that ended on a high note. In these situations, just allow the incident to fade. Don't interfere with the relief your son or daughter is feeling by rebuking them. Thanks to the way you handled the situation, your child has started to learn a very valuable lesson: how to calm himself or her-self down when feeling upset.

More severe meltdowns have their own conse-quences. If you have to spend half an hour calming your preschooler's tantrum, you may have to speed through the rest of your shopping and there might not be time for that quick stop at the toy store or bookstore. Be sure you are very matter-of-fact when you explain these con-sequences—you're not punishing your child's behavior, but the meltdown means that you have to change plans.

If your child broke something or hurt someone, nat-urally there are more serious consequences. If, for exam-ple, Paul had hit his friend when they started arguing about their game, his mom would have separated them, and possibly called Chris's parents to take him home. When Karl broke the bowl, Dad told him, "When Mom gets home, you should tell her right away that you're sorry that you got angry and broke it, and be sure to ask what you can do to make up for breaking it." While they were cleaning up the broken pieces together, he had an-other idea: "You know, that whole set of bowls is getting old and chipped. What if we found some really nice new ones for her birthday present? We could share the cost."

Whatever consequences you decide upon, they must be appropriate and they need to be immediate. Appropri-ate consequences flow naturally from the child's action and are in line with the severity of the offense. Calmly, clearly, and *after having offered your child a choice, and enough time to make the choice, enforce the consequence* of his behavior. For example, if you tell your child that you have to leave the store if the tantrum doesn't stop, then you have no choice—you have to leave the store if the tantrum continues. *You must follow through on every consequence you set, or your child will quickly begin to ignore what you say.* This is true at every age.

There are two bottom lines: first, it's best if the consequences have been *agreed upon ahead of time*; second, you must *always* carry through with consequences, so choose them thoughtfully and be sure that you're going to be in a position to enforce them.

NOTE FROM MOM

THE TOP OF THE REFRIGERATOR

I was chatting with another mom while our toddler girls played together. When they got into a bit of a squabble, the other mom swooped in and yelled, "I'm so tired of you girls fighting. Stop it or that toy is going in the garbage and I'm taking it to the dump!"

This was my first child and I was learning how to parent, so this gave me a good example of what *not* to do: The other mom overreacted, both with her anger and with the severity of the consequence. She also threatened the girls with something she obviously was not going to do.

My husband and I decided that when our children misused their toys—fought over them or left them lying around—we would put the toy on top of the refrigerator until after lunch the next day. "This toy needs a rest (or a better place to stay); it comes down tomorrow after lunch." To a toddler, tomorrow seems a long way off, but on the other hand they know they'll get their toy back. It's a simple consequence, and they know this is always the rule. It's easy to enforce and it's not too harsh.

This also works for children of all ages who leave their belongings strewn throughout the house, although as they get taller you may have to change venues and keep the offending items in your closet until the next day.

6. You're the coach

Coaching is an excellent metaphor for parenting. And good coaching begins long before the actual game. A good coach doesn't try to teach his players new moves during a game; he makes notes of their performance and holds an after-game meeting to discuss how things went and what needs to be worked on during the next practice. In the same way, don't try to explain your children's brain/body imbalance to them while they're in the middle of a meltdown. But as soon as they've calmed down, be sure to help them gain some insight into what triggered this particular meltdown and what they might do to avoid it in the future. For younger children and minor meltdowns, it may be as simple as saying, "You were out in the sun too long, weren't you? That always gets you steamed up. Anytime you start feeling hot, come in and have a nice cool drink to help you cool down."

If your child was extremely rude or hurt someone or did something else serious, spend some time discussing what happened—but first calm yourself down as quickly as you can. Don't wait too long—the situation is naturally winding down and you don't want to prolong it. Make sure your child understands the kind of imbalance that caused his meltdown; discuss how to avoid such an imbalance and how to deal with it *before it escalates*. Talk about what the child did wrong and why you enforced the consequence as you did. Be clear. Be simple. Be concise. *Don't lecture*, because you're only going to have their full attention for a minute or two—that's all a young brain can handle. Your goal is for your children to reflect, without guilt or shame, on what they've done and *why it happened*. You can always offer advice, but kids will learn the most from the incident if they can grasp on their own why their behavior was inappropriate.

Try to develop a style that's the *complete opposite* of "laying down the law" (a punitive means of communication that always meets with resistance and resentment, even if it's not expressed). It also produces immediate and long-term frustration and unhappiness, both for the child and the parent. Good parenting involves inspiring your child to do better and always looking for and reinforcing positive behavior. Never shame or humiliate your child or try to make your child feel guilty. Attempts to control children by making them feel bad about themselves create teenagers and adults who believe that they are bad and must do bad things to get what they need in life. If you want your children to grow up and become loving and productive adults, treat them with love, respect, and appreciation.

Coaching involves being alert and paying attention. As a coach, be alert to intervene when your child is in danger of a meltdown. It's a lot easier to prevent a meltdown than to endure one. Stop whatever you're doing right away and give your child your undivided attention. It might be difficult or inconvenient for you, but usually it isn't impossible. For example, perhaps you're in the middle of cooking dinner and time is tight. You could turn down the burners for a moment, give your child a hug, and say, "I see that you're upset right now [or however the child is feeling], and I want to help you work it out, so as soon as we finish dinner, can we take some time to talk about what's going on?" As soon as dinner is over, thank your child for being patient and then spend some focused time together.

Coaching is a lifelong process. With age you gain experience and wisdom, and you naturally become a better coach. Challenges you meet with one child will help you with the next. And you'll learn from other parents, blogs, books, and articles. There may well be times, however, when you need expert help. If your child continues to have serious meltdowns, it may be a symptom of deeper emotional problems or serious family dysfunctions. In this case, we urge you to consult with a family counselor; your school should be able to help you find a qualified professional.

NOTE FROM MOM

THREE VALUABLE QUESTIONS

Even when dealing with a grown child, *or with yourself*, there are three simple questions that are often the best tools you have to help your child: **deepen his understanding, develop a sense of compassion,** and **improve the child's relationships.**

As soon as your kids are old enough to communicate—through grade school, high school, university, and to the present day—whenever it seems that one of them needs to consider the feelings of another (often, but not necessarily, in the context of their having some responsibility for how the other person was feeling), ask these questions:

1. The feeling question: "How would you feel if this happened to you?"

Listen to what the child says, and relate to it. Perhaps make further suggestions, and talk it through.

2. The thinking question: "What could you do to make the person feel better or to show that you are sorry?"

This teaches your child to be proactive and positive in emotionally challenging situations. Even if circumstances prevent its implementation, your child's *desire and intention* to improve the situation will help him to develop thoughtfulness and compassion.

3. The future question: "What do you think you might do differently next time?"

This question helps kids think about what they could do (or not do!) to encourage **a more positive event** in the future.

CHAPTER 7

THE SIXTH TOOL OF DHARMA PARENTING:
Anticipate and Adapt

REMEMBER THE CONCEPT OF DHARMA? Your dharma is your "path" in life—the style of life that supports your greatest growth, success, happiness, and fulfillment. The dharma of a parent is to help everyone in the family flourish in their own dharma. Whether you are focused on nurturing your child's particular talents or working to ensure that family life moves smoothly through all the changes and adjustments that naturally occur, part of your dharma as a parent is to *anticipate* your family's needs and proactively avoid problems. Despite your best efforts, unexpected events arise and you need to adapt, using your best judgment and creativity to deal with the situation. Here's how "anticipate and adapt" works with the other Dharma Parenting tools:

ANTICIPATE HOW EACH BRAIN/BODY TYPE WILL RESPOND

Once you understand each family member's brain/body type and your own, it's no longer a mystery why different children respond differently to the same situation. You can then take this a step further by anticipating their reactions and planning ahead to keep everyone in balance.

If your budding Vata dancer daughter has an upcoming recital, you know that her schedule will be hectic and she'll inevitably become anxious—and that both of these will further aggravate her Vata. Avoid any potential source of anxiety, allowing plenty of time to do whatever needs to be done without rushing, and keep your Vata child on an even keel by maintaining a balanced, stable routine with plenty of rest.

If your dancer is Pitta, the child will probably enjoy the excitement of the challenging schedule, but if he goes out of balance, your child might also annoy everyone by acting like a prima donna (Pittas, as we've mentioned, love to dominate). Keep them down to earth by maintaining a regular schedule, which includes their usual chores, and be careful not to inflame their Pitta with spicy food.

Kapha dancers will enjoy being part of a dance troupe, but may have trouble adapting to the ever-changing schedule. If there's too much change, they may become stubborn and refuse to budge. Be sure to give your Kapha plenty of advance notice before every new event: when you pick them up from rehearsal, remind them when the next one will be, with more reminders the night before and the morning of. Allow your Kapha extra time to dress, gather his belongings, and get into the car. You might want to mention to the dance teacher— who is probably used to dealing with Vatas and Pittas—that your Kapha needs a little extra attention when a new adjustment is required.

This principle doesn't just apply to special situations. Whenever the family is together, you must take into account how each of the various brain/body types will interact.

Anticipating their interactions is usually pretty easy; the challenge is figuring out how to proactively avert altercations.

For example: What happens when you need to get all your kids out the door at the same time? If it's winter, this can be a major production, with snowsuits, hats, scarves, boots, mittens, not to mention layering! If you start getting everyone ready at the same time, you may be creating an inevitable collision: Your little Vata will be running out the door impatiently before his Kapha sister has one boot on. Your efficient Pitta will, meanwhile, be all suited up . . . and get overheated in all that outdoor gear. Anticipate the situation by reminding your Kapha child at breakfast, then an hour, and then half an hour, and then fifteen minutes before it's time to leave! Pile each child's gear next to him and get each of them started, then tell your Pitta child to get ready and organize everything to take to the car. Then you can make sure your Vata child actually puts on all the necessary warm clothes before heading out the door.

Another common occasion for brain/body type collisions is mealtime: the food that balances one type may aggravate another. Anticipate such collisions with thoughtful menu planning. If the forecast calls for cold, wet weather, leave cold, heavy foods off the menu to avoid aggravating your family's Kapha tendencies. If one family member faces a challenge—whether it's the first day of preschool or college entrance exams—build the menu around the needs of that person's brain/body type to help keep him in balance at this critical time.

ANTICIPATE HEALING YOURSELF

You are the primary support system for your family, so whenever extra demands are placed on any one family member, some of that extra load will naturally shift over to you. It's essential that you anticipate how to keep yourself rested, fresh, and in good balance. If you're going to be on taxi duty all weekend, pack water (in winter, your favorite hot beverage) and nutritious snacks for yourself, not just for your children. If your schedule is going to be hectic next week, call on *your* support system (or create one) to help you get additional rest over the weekend. Look ahead and see if you can off-load some of your regular duties. For example, if you're in charge of meals, this may be the time to call in an alternate chef or to switch to frozen pizza or your favorite takeout for a couple of evenings. You can let some of your weekly chores slide; ask one of your older children to add the laundry to his to-do list.

If you meditate, be sure to fit in that all-important renewal time twice a day. This is a good moment to remember that it really is possible (though perhaps not ideal) for you to meditate *anywhere*. Parents of busy offspring often find themselves meditating in the car while waiting for a rehearsal to end, or between tennis matches. Anticipate the situation by being on the lookout for a quiet and more or less private place to meditate—a shady parking place or a chair in a nearby library.

ANTICIPATE WHEN YOUR KIDS WILL NEED EXTRA ATTENTION AND APPRECIATION

If someone has an important exam or surgery (wisdom teeth, anyone?), or maybe an out-of-town trip or an upcoming performance, naturally that child needs more attention. A situation can arise if one child is ill for very long. What about the rest of the family? Anticipate that they may feel a bit neglected if you have to give most of your time and attention to one child. While you're rushing around attending to the very specific needs of one child, take time to prepare some favorite snacks and read the other kids a second bedtime story. If the schedule gets truly chaotic, you can at least give them a few words of sincere appreciation and a hug. Check in with your spouse, too—with so many extra parenting duties, you'll both appreciate a little additional communication and support.

The big events are easy to anticipate, but children often feel challenged by day-to-day happenings as well. For example, a Kapha child who's had extensive and difficult dental work may remember the experience for many years (that excellent Kapha memory isn't always a blessing) and still be nervous about going to the dentist in his teens. Anticipating this upcoming stress, you will want to give your child some extra attention beforehand, along with extra hugs and support en route.

ANTICIPATE CHANGES IN THE ROUTINE

Routines help everyone automatically anticipate what needs to be done. Do I want a bedtime story? My routine tells me that I should start my bath at seven fifteen. Do I need to catch the school bus at seven thirty? My routine gets me out of bed at six forty-five so I have time for breakfast.

But there are times when routines seem to fly out the window. Family vacation is one of those times. It's a great opportunity to enjoy new places and spend time together, but it can be incredibly challenging for parents to keep everyone occupied and balanced so the trip isn't spoiled by meltdowns.

Here's how Keith's daughter-in-law, Danielle, the mother of three kids, ages seven months and six and seven years, anticipated the family's needs proactively on a long car vacation. (Could Danielle possibly be a predominantly Pitta brain/body type?)

*I wanted to limit movie, computer, and electronic
game time. For each child, I made a binder and
printed out some fun games from the Internet: designs
and pictures to color, mazes, crossword and word-find
puzzles, car bingo. I also printed out a map, which
was the first page in each binder. I included coloring
pencils and stickers they could use to decorate the
binder covers. My husband made a summer music
folder on his cell phone so we could hear our favorite
songs in the car. Books on tape are also popular, but
our kids prefer singing out loud! From Iowa to
Michigan, the kids did not ask once for a movie.*

*I was hoping that our new baby would sleep most
of the time, and when she was awake, she would be
entertained by the kids in the backseat because her car
seat faced them. And I was right!*

*Before we left I introduced the older kids to an old
digital camera and to our already existing family
website. I showed them how to open and close the
camera, how to charge its battery, how to delete pictures, and how to upload them onto the computer. I
made a folder called "Michigan" on the laptop we
were planning to bring along. Our family website is
really simple, drag-and-drop. I sent an e-mail to rel-
atives and friends inviting them to visit the website,
where the kids would post pictures to show where we
were going and what we did. Everyone could visit it
and comment on the pictures and blog. The kids became enthusiastic and were inspired to continue for
the whole week.*

*I also prepared snack bags with special snacks: gra-
nola bars, fruit leather, and applesauce in a cup*

(which they can drink if they poke a straw in the cup—less mess in the car). On each snack bag I printed: "Do not open until," so we could write in either the time or a town along the way. I also added some small toys to the snack bags, and we used the empty bags for garbage. The kids could look on their maps to see where we were or check the clock to see whether it was snack time.

It was a fun trip, with good memories, and our kids have stories and pictures to enjoy on our website for another year. (See gojindy.com.)

A lot of work? Yes, but because Danielle anticipated her children's needs so well, she could enjoy the vacation along with her family. It would have been much more work if the children had been restless and irritable, demanding extra attention in the middle of the car trip.

Suppose you're going to a family event, such as a wedding. The kids may not know the bride or groom, and all the activities are designed for adults. Anticipate how to keep your children happy and occupied. You don't have to limit yourself to providing games or other recreation; if you can figure out how the kids can help with the preparations (without getting in everyone's way), they will feel more involved and useful. Include their cousins, and all the parents will be singing your praises.

ANTICIPATE MELTDOWNS

Remember Paul, Valerie, and Karl from chapter 6? Let's consider how their parents might have anticipated—and therefore, prevented—their meltdowns.

First, Paul: It was a hot day, and with her Pitta son playing out in the sun, Mom might easily have anticipated that tempers would fly if Paul and his friend got overheated. With attention and anticipation, she could have figured out how long they could play peacefully in the heat, and well *before* the critical point, dispense a cooling agent: popsicles, root beer floats, or—better yet—a pair of loaded water guns or buckets of water to start a wild water battle. If she miscalculated the boy's heat exposure and they started to melt down, she would have had the cold treats or the full water weapons ready for deployment. After this welcome interruption, it would then be easy to move them to a cooler venue, indoors to watch a movie or play a game or off to the swimming pool.

Valerie's Vata meltdown was a little harder to anticipate. Her parents probably were not aware of the e-mail requesting her to choose her seminar class. Mom and Dad might, however, have anticipated that Valerie's Vata brain/body type would predispose her to be anxious about the many decisions she was going to have to make starting college. Even before she had to choose which college to attend, they could help her develop a decision-making protocol that works for her—including Internet research, creating lists of pros and cons, and discussing options with her parents and with her high school counselor. An established routine for making decisions will give Valerie a sense of stability and control to help her work through all her upcoming life-shaping decisions.

Karl's dad helped keep him in balance by praising his performance during the game, but that wasn't enough to head off a meltdown. After the game, Dad might have anticipated that Karl, as a Kapha brain/body type, would need extra time to recover from the disappointment of being shifted to first base and then losing the game. Father and son could have had an after-game snack together, before Karl was plunged back into the maelstrom of a houseful of younger brothers and sisters. Spending time alone with Dad would also have given Karl some extra attention, which helps any brain/body type, of any age, feel more settled and confident.

ANTICIPATE AND ADAPT

The ability to anticipate comes from understanding and using all of the Dharma Parenting tools, plus the basic knowledge of brain development described in section 2. Once you realize that your children's abilities and reactions are different from yours because their brain/body types and levels of brain development are different, you can understand that they are truly doing the best they can with the abilities they have. If they're slow or irritable or restless, they aren't doing it to annoy you; it's their built-in response to the situation. They're not less intelligent than you, and their reactions are just as valid as yours; they are, however, younger and have different brain/body types. When you respect your children as full human beings, they learn to respect themselves and to respect you. Establishing this mutual respect is the best proactive tool any parent can have to avert most problems and constructively solve the rest.

Being proactive and anticipating possible scenarios is your first and best choice, but when unexpected events come up you need to *adapt*. You're the expert on how to raise your child, and ultimately you know what's best for your child, not based on logic, rules, and prescriptions, but based on feeling, intuition, trust, and your love. You always have the freedom to adapt—to do what is needed at the moment. More than anyone else on earth, you know who your child is. Enhance this knowledge by learning as much as you can about your child's brain/body type. And make sure that your own brain stays alert and rested so you can always appreciate and pay *real* attention to your child.

The book *How to Talk So Kids Will Listen & Listen So Kids Will Talk*, by Adele Faber and Elaine Mazlish, gives an excellent example of a parent adapting brilliantly. A six-year-old boy had a condition that required him to wear a patch over his right eye for six months. The patch had to be worn every day for four hours. The boy was uncomfortable and told his mom that he couldn't see very well when he wore the patch and that it hurt him. The mother acknowledged his feelings but insisted he wear the patch.

Her son continued to complain and was growing more and more irritated. After a week, she was at her wit's end, and said that she would wear the patch to experience what it was like. Much to her surprise, within twenty minutes she had a terrible headache. She lost depth perception and had trouble even opening up a cupboard. She quickly took her son to their optometrist and spoke with him about the experience. From then on the boy wore the patch to school every day with no argument. His sight completely improved, and he didn't even have to wear glasses.

Notice that the mother did not take an authoritative stance and say, "Wear it!" She listened to her child and respected his feelings. She adapted to this situation, following her own judgment and intuition. Her willingness to wear the patch herself reconciled her son to wearing it. The point of this story is that we may *think* that we understand what our child is going through, but we don't—unless we ourselves "walk a mile in the other's shoes." Giving our child *empathetic attention* must always be one of our very highest parenting priorities.

DHARMA PARENTING TOOLS FOR FOUR MAIN AGE GROUPS

CHAPTER 8

DHARMA PARENTING TOOLS:
The First Years of Life, Zero to Three

NEURAL EXUBERANCE

The amazing advances in the first three years of your child's life are more complex and fascinating to watch than any TV show. During this short period, your baby's brain cells create *twenty-four million neural connections every minute.* That's not a typo: twenty-four million. Aptly this remarkable process is called "neural exuberance."

Imagine buying a computer and receiving a boxful of parts; all the necessary electronics are there but they must be wired together before you can use it. The situation is similar to the state of your baby's brain at birth: all the neurons are there, one hundred billion of them—as many as you have now—but they're not yet connected. This is why your infant does not at first "see" a mom, dad, sister, or brother. The newborn brain lacks the neural connections necessary to generate an integrated image of a whole person—with head, neck, shoulders, and body. It can only register individual impressions of individual bits of light and color. The newborn brain also possesses the brain cells to hear each individual sound, but again it lacks the connections to link impulses of sound together into words or melodies. Neurons must learn to fire together through *repetition* in order to gradually become wired together and form specific networks. As these neural networks develop, your baby begins to discern familiar faces and voices—Mom's face, Dad's voice.

You can actually observe your baby "training" his brain. Watch as the child waves a toy back and forth in front of its eyes. This is a sort of rehearsal in which the same groups of neurons fire together again and again, creating neural pathways and networks that allow the baby to start recognizing and tracking familiar objects.

By the end of the first three years, each brain cell may be connected to a thousand other brain cells—one hundred trillion possible connections, more than the number of stars in the universe. There are so many connections that a three-year-old's cortex—the surface layer of the brain where most of the processing occurs—is twice as thick as yours! And as the connections increase over these years, you can witness your child's hearing, sight, movement, and speech improving.

Another important process occurs at the same time. A thin layer of fat, called "myelin," starts wrapping around the connections within the sensory areas of the brain and the motor system. This protective coating does two things: It insulates the neurons from interference, and it speeds the flow of information by twenty times. With faster information flow, the infant can see an object moving through space as a whole, rather than a collection of disconnected colors and edges—it's like watching a high-definition movie rather than a film from the early 1900s.

THINKING AND LEARNING

From birth to three years, your baby's mental world goes through major transformations. In the first few months the infant is overwhelmed by fragmented and disconnected sensory experiences. And the behavior of newborns reflects this: They don't interact much with the world because they are not fully equipped to make sense of it. They randomly wave their arms and legs around and grasp anything put into their hands. But after three or four months, they begin to put these unthinking reflexes together: they grasp a rattle and wave it in front of their eyes on purpose, or bring it to their mouth and suck on it. A month or so later, they begin to observe the world around them and notice that they can actually change that world. When they drop a toy from their high chair, they now expect you to pick it up—and then laugh with glee when they drop it again. Your baby does not yet have the brain connections to make a *conscious* link between what they do and the consequences of that action—they don't consciously think, "It would be really fun to make Dad pick up my rattle seven times in a row." They're simply observing that certain of their actions have interesting and repeatable effects.

At one year, the brain can knit sensory input together to create dazzling shapes and sounds that completely transfix the child. And near the end of the first year, children begin to engage in "goal-directed behavior"; in other words, they begin to understand how they can make something happen. For example, rather than crawling over to a toy sitting in a wagon, a one-year-old might pull the wagon toward himself. Listen to your child's laughter as he begins to exercise this newfound relationship. Your child is beginning to learn that specific behavior creates certain consequences. Your son or daughter is learning to control the environment in order to fulfill a desire.

Another important change in perception is the development of "object permanence," which occurs at about the same time. During the first nine months of life, an object (or person) only exists for infants while they can actually see it; when it's no longer in sight, it no longer exists for them. Each time they see that favorite toy again, it's as if it has magically come into being, and there's an expression of wonder and delight on their faces. If you hide a toy from children of this age, they won't look for it, because they don't yet have the brain circuits needed to create an image of something when it's not in front of their eyes. At around nine months, however, children will search for the toy, because they have a picture of it in their mind. This is object permanence.

Object permanence is the basis for playing the game of peekaboo. When we place a blanket over a child's head, the world disappears. For a baby who's less than nine months old, this is quite frightening. But after nine months, it becomes exhilarating. The nine-month-old has some degree of confidence that the world still exists, even when he cannot see it. Notice the child's joyful thrill when you remove the blanket. It's as if she is saying, "Yes! I was right, and isn't the world wonderful!"

Your child's social life also undergoes great transformations in the period from birth to three years. After the first few months, babies begin to recognize speech and to babble to themselves, which is practice for speaking. From one to one and a half years, they begin to play with other children and to share toys. They also listen closely to adult talk. By two or three years, the child develops language, begins to label objects, and begins to imagine what might happen. This is the beginning of creative play—a box can be a spaceship, a monster, or a restaurant. At this point children are also beginning to use sentences to communicate their feelings.

Of course, different children experience these milestones at different ages, and you will notice other accomplishments during these dynamic years. Treasure this time. Your child will never again change so much in such a short period. You may want to keep track of their growth in a notebook or on your phone; you can also buy special calendars with stickers for first-year growth milestones. We warn you, though, if you create one of these calendars for your first child, be sure to do the same for the others, or they'll certainly ask, "Where's *my* calendar?"

NOTE FROM MOM

STROLLER OR PACK?

We've made the point that infants do not yet possess "object permanence." If they can't see something, it doesn't exist for them. Imagine that you are a baby in a stroller, seated facing forward: You can't see your parents (for all you know you're alone in the world). Nobody talks to you because you're several feet away and they can't look you in the face. Also, you're about twenty inches from the ground, with the world whizzing by—mostly knees and car doors and the lower shelves in stores. If you're less than five months old, you don't even have depth perception yet. The world as seen from a stroller creates feelings of isolation, and doesn't make much sense.

In contrast, imagine that you're an infant in a front carrier: You can see, hear, feel, and smell your parent or caretaker. You're warm and cuddled, so you feel loved and secure. If you're sleepy, you can snuggle in and nap. Your adult naturally talks to you because you're right there in front of him. And if you're feeling confident and exuberant, you can always face outward and enjoy the world from a perspective where you can see people's faces.

When you (the baby) get bigger and move to a backpack, you really become part of the action. You can even see over people's heads. Not to mention grabbing your parent's hair, poking your knees in their ribs, and "talking" to them. Now you feel very much like your parent's buddy, a great feeling for any child.

APPLYING DHARMA PARENTING TOOLS DURING THE FIRST THREE YEARS

TOOL 1: DISCOVER YOUR CHILD'S BRAIN/BODY TYPE

During the first few months, you can identify your child's body type—one aspect of their brain/body type—by observing his temperament, body structure, and reactions. The child who throws off blankets, is impatient, and reacts strongly to experiences is probably a Pitta type. The Kapha type is generally placid and loves to sleep. The Vata type is highly sensitive and often restless; their bodies are usually long and thin or small and delicate.

Knowing your infant's body type helps you keep your child in balance by adjusting baby's diet and activities. Until a child starts to eat solid food, diet is easy to control. Keep in mind that a breast-fed baby is affected by its mother's diet—for example, the mom of a Pitta infant would want to avoid eating lots of spicy food. When your child begins to eat new foods, refer to the diet suggestions for each of the body types discussed in chapter 1.

As babies enter the toddler stage, it's important to tailor their activities to their particular physiology in order to keep them in good balance. For example, make sure that your Vata child has a steady routine with plenty of creative outlets and activity, but not too much exertion. Typically, Pitta children will do best with lots of purposeful play—for example, building with Legos or learning a new skill can keep them absorbed for hours. They also love to compete. Keep them out of the heat, however, and encourage them to learn to swim. Kapha children are generally easygoing; your main challenge will probably be to stimulate them toward healthy physical activity.

The second aspect of brain/body types is the level of brain development. Being alert to your children's changing levels of brain development enables you to adjust your parenting to their current abilities—you won't ask for more than their brains can handle, and you won't hold them back by not engaging them enough.

TOOL 2: HEAL YOURSELF

> *Katie sits sobbing at the kitchen table, her head in her arms. Her two-month-old daughter, Ellie, has been crying for hours. No matter what Katie does, the baby keeps screaming at the top of her lungs. Katie is horrified to find herself yelling, "Will you please shut up for five freaking minutes!"*
>
> *Katie is a single mom weighed down by the endless physical, emotional, and financial demands of being a parent. Both she and baby Ellie are Vata brain/body types, so they both are easily tired and upset, and they*

> *haven't established set routines. Katie is hesitant to call*
> *on her family and friends for support, telling herself*
> *that she made her choices and she's responsible for fol-*
> *lowing through with them. But now she realizes that*
> *she's at the end of her rope and really needs support.*
>   *Wearily, she picks up the phone to call her mom.*
> *Next, she decides, I'll call my brother and my best*
> *friend. I've got to get some help before I end up hurt-*
> *ing Ellie. The family told me that they care; I sure*
> *hope they mean it.*

Your family and friends are often eager to help out, although their own individual brain/body types will determine
how they might best help. Katie's mom is a Kapha type. She's
naturally sweet and soothing, which helps calm both Ellie
and Katie. As soon as she walks through the door, Katie immediately feels her stability. Grandma holds the infant close
and sings to her. The Kapha qualities of groundedness and
evenness help to balance the Vata baby. After Ellie finally falls
asleep in Grandma's arms, Katie and her mom set up a schedule for Grandma to come over a couple days a week to help,
not just with the baby, but with the housework and laundry
too. This will allow Katie to get badly needed rest and, just as
important, it will relieve some of her anxiety and give her a
chance to learn a few parenting skills from her mother.

Katie's brother, Pete, is also a Vata type, so he knows that
Vata types like change. He offers to devote his Saturday
mornings to taking Katie and Ellie to do the grocery shopping, then out to lunch and a fun excursion. Pete is engaged
to be married and tells Katie that this is great preparation for
when he'll someday be a dad. His natural flair and high energy always cheer Katie up and distract her from her worries.

Katie's best friend, Janet, is a Pitta type, and she offers to help Katie get more organized. She comes over early Sunday evening so they can cook a gourmet meal together, like they used to when they shared an apartment, then she helps Katie figure out her priorities for work and baby care.

When your baby is young it can be difficult (if not impossible) to find time to heal yourself; you're a parent 24-7 and at any moment of the day or night your child might need you. This can be especially challenging if you're a perfectionist. This is a good time to learn how to compromise, and get comfortable with the reality that *it's okay just to accomplish the necessary things*, because that's all you may have time for during your baby's first year. If your family is fed and safe (with moderately clean clothes), everything else can wait. Eventually you'll manage to fit in laundry and vacuuming. Just be sure to get help from those around you—your partner, friends, and family, or a trusted babysitter or nanny if you can afford it. And wouldn't a housekeeper be heaven! Let them look after the baby for a while so you can get much-needed and well-deserved rest. Even thirty to forty-five minutes a day of "me" time can give you the second wind you need to get through the day. If you have a meditation practice, seize the opportunity to meditate the minute your baby falls asleep in your lap, or when your toddler becomes absorbed with books or blocks. Don't be surprised or upset when your meditation is interrupted—*because it will be.* The good news is that you'll still feel at least somewhat renewed and energized afterward.

What if you don't have family or friends you can call on? Every community has parent support services designed to help you. Check with your local school district, church, or department of human services. Or try an Internet search for your city's name and "parent support"—you may be surprised how many options there are. Once your baby starts walking, try one of the parent-and-child playgroups organized by your YMCA, city recreation department, or local college. This is a great way to connect with other parents and start creating your own support network.

TOOL 3: ATTENTION AND APPRECIATION

A newborn naturally captures all your attention, and rightfully so. This miraculous human being is not only fascinating but needs constant care because he is completely dependent on you for *everything*. As your baby develops, he may need less attention to survive, *but need more attention to be able to thrive*. Start a habit at this early age of *paying full attention* to your child whenever you can. If he asks you a question, stop what you're doing and offer your undivided attention. When you're waiting for the doctor or the dentist, don't just ignore your child while you text or catch up on some work—turn the enforced waiting period into quality time *with* your child. Those books and toys are in the waiting room for a reason. And if your child's attention becomes absorbed in sharing some quiet activity with you, he will be distracted from any anxiety about the doctor or dentist visit. Of course, there may be times when you can't avoid multitasking, especially if you have more than one child, but undivided attention is a gift that will be repaid many times over as your child grows up feeling secure and cherished.

Understanding the basics of your baby's brain development will also allow you to implement the second part of this tool, appreciation. Growth is sometimes obvious: babies start to crawl, then walk, then run. It's harder to discern the inner aspects of development, such as an infant's grasp of depth perception or a toddler's understanding of past and future.

Refer to the chart below for a general idea of a typical developmental timetable. As we often point out, every child develops differently, which you'll certainly notice if you have children with different brain/body types. Vata babies tend to

0–8 months	Coordination: Progress from lifting up their heads to rolling over and then crawling.
	Perception: Depth perception at five months; can focus across the room at eight months.
	Communication: Begin to babble and talk to themselves.
	Socialization: Progress from passive looking to intentional social interactions through eye contact, arm or leg movements, and cuddling.
8–18 months	Coordination: Progress from pulling themselves up to stand, to cruising while holding on to you or the furniture, to walking.
	Perception: Recognize themselves in a mirror; develop object permanence (this is the time to play peekaboo).
	Communication: Respond to their name.
	Socialization: Begin establishing relationships with other children by playing and sharing; listen closely to adult talk.
18–36 months	Coordination: Walk up and down stairs; stand on one foot.
	Perception: Understand the concept of past and future.
	Communication: Use sentences to communicate feelings; enjoy stories and picture books.
	Socialization: Demonstrate pride and pleasure when something is accomplished, and embarrassment when they make a mistake.
	Creative play: Use an object to represent something else (a bowl is a hat).

develop new skills quickly but then forget them the next day and regain them the day after. You can help by gently reminding and patiently helping them along. Pitta types are usually very focused—you can almost see their brains working away to master a new skill. But watch out for signs of frustration if they don't progress as fast as they'd like. Kapha types are more laid-back and may develop many skills later than average, but don't worry—once they've figured something out, they'll remember it forever. Kaphas can be very stubborn about wanting to do things for themselves, and it's good to respect this by allowing extra time for their slow-paced shoelace tying and zippering.

It's important that you appreciate the level of your child's development so your expectations match his abilities. For example, no matter how carefully you toss the ball to your eighteen-month-old, he can't catch it because this level of coordination will not be reached for another couple of years. You don't want to err in the other direction either, by not giving your child appropriate opportunities to grow. When your two-year-old starts struggling with buttons, do not insist on dressing him because it's faster and you do a better job. Allow extra time for kids to wriggle those stubborn buttons into their buttonholes, and let them proudly wear the shirt they just buttoned, no matter how crooked it is. Show your kids that you appreciate their newfound abilities by *giving them time* to figure things out and to practice. As we've mentioned, their neurons are not yet myelinated, so electrical signals travel more slowly in their brains than in yours. You can see for yourself that young children simply do not think as quickly as adults. They need plenty of time to think things through so that their neural pathways can develop fully.

As children's brains develop and their abilities grow, it's also important that you begin to treat them like the thinking people they're becoming. Start letting them participate in decisions that directly affect them: "Would you like your doll or your bear?" "It's a little windy today. Would you like to wear your blue coat or your red sweater?" "We need to go to the grocery store and the library. Which one should we do first?" Showing respect for their opinions not only keeps your relationship smooth now, but it's great practice for the increasingly important decisions they will be making as they get older.

Nurturing Communication Skills

Crying is a newborn's primary means of communication. If only they could put their emotions and sensations into words! They cry and gesture to try to tell us how they feel, but we can't always figure it out—so their crying escalates. Don't just put them down and let them cry themselves to sleep: at this moment, when they're so unhappy and frustrated, they need the comfort of your warmth and your voice more than ever. Your child, no matter how young, is a person too.

As your child grows, continue to listen and respond to his needs. Parents should try to set aside a regular time—maybe before nap time or bedtime—to spend some quiet moments talking with the child. Your attention will pay off many times over as your toddler becomes a child, then an adolescent, a teen, and an adult.

When you're speaking to your baby or preschooler, remember that he can only understand concrete ideas. The brain connections needed to be able to think abstractly or logically simply do not yet exist. Concrete nouns and verbs such as "couch" and "jump" can be easily understood, but negatives are too abstract to grasp at this age. So if you tell your three-year-old, "Don't jump on the couch," the only words the child will really understand are "jump" and "couch"—not the actual message you're trying to get across. Rather than abstract negatives, give your child clear directives: "Please get off the couch," or "The couch is for sitting; the floor is for jumping!" If your children are playing too loudly, in a dentist's waiting room, for instance, don't just tell them, "Stop that!" They actually won't know *what* to stop—moving the toy car? making the loud vrooming noise? laughing? Be more specific and to the point so that they can understand: "Please be quieter" or just make a gentle "Shhhhh." Concepts like right and wrong, good and bad, are also far too abstract for young children to understand. The admonition "Be good!" doesn't mean anything to a young child. But if you're concrete and specific, not only will you be able to communicate, you will also help your child's reasoning power to develop.

TOOL 4: ROUTINES

One of your important tasks during the first three years of your child's life is to establish routines, especially mealtime and bedtime routines that are suited to your baby's brain/body type. A third routine is "getting out" the door. As we discussed, you have to plan ahead, because it takes a lot of organization to get babies and toddlers ready to leave: bottles, favorite toys, snacks, snowsuits, hats, sunblock—no matter what the season, there are lots of accessories to bring along. When your kids get old enough, allow time for them to try to put on their own clothes. Of course, this will take a lot longer in the beginning, but it will pay off when they become self-sufficient thanks to all their practice.

Set Up Eating Routines

> *Distraught, Linda looks down at her wailing six-week-old daughter, Megan. "Oh, little bunny, what am I going to do with you? You have to eat! Please, please," she begs, "have a little more."*
>
> *Megan's a very fussy eater, and even though she's often hungry, she only takes a small amount while breast-feeding. Linda has noticed that her daughter is especially unhappy in the afternoons between three and five. And she's worried because Megan isn't gaining weight like her brother and sister did. With two older kids to care for and a husband who's often away on business, Linda is feeling badly stressed. She knows that she needs relief, but what can she do?*

Many babies have an uncomfortable period that regularly occurs in the late afternoon or evening, and this is especially true for Vata babies like Megan. Vatas need to eat frequently, in a quiet and pleasant environment, without distractions, and with Mom's *full attention*. We encourage you to do everything possible, for your child's sake and your own, to be comfortable and feel as good as you can: eat well and get extra rest and mild exercise. While your infant is nursing, pamper yourself and your child with lovely music and aroma oil. As your Vata baby gets older and transitions to solid food, keep the routine of *small, frequent meals in a settled environment*.

If Megan were a Kapha or a Pitta brain/body type, Linda would probably have far less to worry about. Both types enjoy their meals, although the Pitta type tends to be more focused on food and quite a bit more demanding than the laid-back, contented Kapha type.

Setting Up Sleep Routines

Which sleep strategy is best for your baby? Well, that depends on your child's body type and stage of brain development. If your infant is a Kapha brain/body type, you may not understand the fuss other parents make about getting their babies to sleep. Give the baby some warm milk, burp him, and the child falls asleep in your arms within a few minutes; then when you lay the baby down, he sleeps most of the night. Nevertheless, even with a Kapha child, it's good to set up a regular bedtime routine right away. As the child gets older he may start to stubbornly resist bedtime. This simply means that your intelligent offspring has figured out that after the book is read, Mommy or Daddy is going to leave the room. Try to maintain a familiar routine, altering it slightly because "now you're getting to be so big and strong." Kapha brain/body types are especially soothed by physical contact, so extra cuddles may do the trick.

If your baby is a Vata brain/body type, you'll soon be adding your own stories to the saga of sleep challenges. First they want a little milk; then they're restless and take a long time to fall asleep. No matter how gently you lay them down, they're very likely to wake back up. If their tummy isn't full, they wake up for more milk several times a night. Their sleep problems simply reflect how their physiology is functioning; please don't let grandparents or aunts or *anyone* label them as bad or difficult because they have trouble sleeping. Vata brain/body types will probably always take longer to fall asleep and be more easily disturbed than other children; this may hold true even when they're adults. For Vatas, a quiet, subdued, and pleasant bedtime environment is essential. They will also be sensitive to your agitation if you're upset with them, so keep firmly in mind that their sleeplessness is not their fault. If you become impatient—and sooner or later, who can avoid it?—hand them over to your spouse or partner. As they grow older, be sure to maintain the same soothing bedtime routine, because its familiarity will help lull them to sleep. Vata brain/body types love choices, so you could let them decide whether they want a story first or a song, or let them participate in telling the story.

Pitta brain/body types are a little easier as infants, and if you keep them in a quiet environment so they're not overstimulated, they'll usually settle down. Try to avoid disturbances—Pitta kids will wake up instantly to see what's going on. It's fun to watch a Pitta baby fall asleep: they try to keep their eyes open as long as possible because the world is so fascinating, and when at last sleep overtakes them, their eyes may snap shut. Their strong digestion means they may wake up hungry in the middle of the night. As they get older, they might resist going to bed because they don't want to end the day until they've figured out how the universe functions. Entice them by letting them look at picture books or play with simple puzzles in bed. But be careful not to raise any questions because their intellect will click on and it'll take even more time to get them to settle down again.

TOOL 5: MANAGE MELTDOWNS

Your three-month-old is crying harder and harder, and you've tried everything—food, a diaper change, burping, blankets—and you're getting frantic. Is your baby having a meltdown? Not really. Your child is just letting you know how very uncomfortable he is—and will keep on telling you until you can fix it. You must use everything you know about your child as well as your intuition to figure out what's wrong and how to correct it. Keep using this approach as the child gets closer to the "terrible twos" (which can occur later, though rarely earlier).

Back to neural exuberance: For over two years, your child's brain has been creating twenty-four million new connections *every minute*. By the age of three, the child's brain will have the most connections it will ever have. And because of these dramatic brain changes, two-year-olds are undergoing jumps in physical coordination and in intellectual, social, and emotional changes. Their vocabularies are growing, and they're eager to do things on their own. They are also beginning to have a sense of past and future, and they expect and count on certain things to occur. When something different happens, their world comes tumbling down. Welcome to the terrible twos.

> *Nancy is very concerned about her two-year-old son. Jayden had always been a happy, even-tempered little boy, but recently his emotions have been getting out of control.*
>
> *A typical example occurred one day last week when Nancy planned to take Jayden to the park to feed the ducks. The boy was very pleased and excited about it and had been looking forward to it for several days. Unfortunately, right before they left the house, Nancy got a call that the deadline for one of her part-time editing jobs had been pushed up and it had to be finished by the next morning. There was nothing she could do but to put off the outing. Jayden could neither understand nor accept the change in plans, and responded by screaming loudly and throwing himself on the ground. Half an hour later, he was still going strong.*
>
> *Nancy's at her wit's end. She and her husband*

*have even been thinking about taking Jayden to a
doctor or a child psychologist.*

The most important thing for Nancy to know is that this
really is *not* abnormal behavior for a two-year-old child. At
this age, kids are beginning to be able to anticipate events, so
they expect and count on certain things to occur. They completely identify with the picture they've built up in their
minds, and if it doesn't happen, their sense of self is shattered.
This is why Jayden was so deeply disappointed, confused, and
frustrated when he didn't get to feed the ducks.

The six C's will help you deal with terrible twos' meltdowns.
Let's summarize the key steps for Nancy:

- **Check** in with yourself and your child

  Not only is Nancy under pressure to finish her
  editing job, but her son is now kicking and screaming on the floor. She knows that she needs to stay
  calm and deal with the situation rationally. It
  would help if she could keep in mind that the terrible twos are *more terrible for the two-year-old* than
  for the parent. Jayden isn't throwing this tantrum
  in order to manipulate her. He was so completely
  invested in going to feed the ducks that his world is
  shattered. Understanding this should help Nancy
  be sympathetic rather than punitive.

- **Comfort** your child

  Jayden feels confused and threatened. He needs
  to know that everything will be all right and that
  his mom is there to help and support him. He's so

agitated that Nancy may not be able to hug him initially, but she can stay nearby and rub his back or hold his hand so that he knows she's there.

- **Change** your child's brain state

   This is a good time for Nancy to use a "brain trick." Deep in the brain, our hippocampus is always alert for novel sensory information. If the hippocampus detects a radically new stimulus, it directs full attention to the new experience. Nancy can put this bit of knowledge to use by speaking quietly and slowly. Her screaming son will soon stop and ask, "What did you say?" Mom's quiet speech is such a contrast to Jayden's screaming that his hippocampus will judge it to be more important than his tantrum and redirect Jayden's attention to what she's saying.

- Offer **choices**

   Once Jayden has cooled down a bit, Nancy can begin to give him some concrete choices: "After lunch tomorrow when we go feed the ducks, what kind of bread shall we take them?" or "Which duck will you feed first—the brown one you fed last time or that little one with the blue head?" These are attractive ideas, and Jayden will finish cooling down as he considers each one carefully. His mind is now engaged rather than disturbed by raging emotions.

- Enforce **consequences**

   In Jayden's perception, his small world has just turned upside down. And there might be some natural consequences—has he broken a toy? Then he won't be able to play with it anymore. In this case, Nancy doesn't feel the need to create consequences; this was simply a two-year-old storm that she and Jayden had to ride out. His mother's loving, soothing attitude will help Jayden learn to calm himself as his brain develops and his world expands.

- You're the **coach**

    Nancy dealt with Jayden's meltdown effectively because she acted as a coach, trying to help him, *not* as a "boss" whose job it is to lay down the law. She's learned an essential parenting lesson: *Your role is to be a loving and knowledgeable parent who helps your child cope with inner feelings, deal with disappointment, and develop independence.*

TOOL 6: ANTICIPATE AND ADAPT

As the parent of a newborn, you can be overwhelmed by everything you need to learn, and by the responsibility of making good choices for this precious new human being. There are so many new skills to master, so many new routines to figure out. If you're aware of your child's pattern of development over the next few years, you'll be preparing a smoother parenting path for yourself.

For instance, as babies become toddlers and then preschoolers, they begin to figure things out on their own and express their own opinions. This is the point when you need to stop treating your son or daughter like a powerless baby and start relating to your child as a thinking human being. Since you probably won't be able to discern the exact moment this magical transformation takes place, play it safe by anticipating it long before it happens. Think about Tom and Laura back in chapter 4: They were letting their baby "choose" what to wear when she was five months old. They anticipated that she would soon be able to make decisions like these and figured that she might as well start practicing early.

Of course, you have to adapt to your child's abilities. If your son or daughter is a Pitta, he will probably love the opportunity to make decisions, but Vata and Kapha brain/body types may have trouble if you introduce too many choices too early. If your child seems at all confused when you offer several choices or ask his opinion, either simplify the choices or wait a couple of weeks and try again.

"Adapt" is a one-word slogan for parenting young children. Every bit of advice you receive and every fact you learn about their development must be adapted to your child's brain/body type and level of development. You must also adapt your thinking and actions to your child's current needs, discarding the routines that worked last week and adapting them to the new person your child has become this week.

An example of anticipating/adapting is the need to childproof the home. Electrical outlets, sharp corners, and vases that tip and break need to be secured. Children who are allowed to explore a safe environment grow with more inner motivation, curiosity, and openness to try new things. Consider the following story:

CHILDPROOFING THE HOME

"What's that racket?" Brooke asks her husband, Jeremy, as they're straightening up the living room. Running into the kitchen, Jeremy finds their one-year-old son, Ethan, pulling everything out of the re-

*cycling bin and throwing cans and bottles against the
wall with great energy.*

*Ethan is interested in, and wants to gets his hands
on, everything—magazines on the living room coffee
table, the garbage, the contents of closets, even the lit-
ter in the cat's box!*

The boy is strong willed and fast moving, and his parents
understand that they must be proactive before their son's behavior results in a horrible mess or—worse—an accident.
They decide to spend the afternoon doing a better job of
childproofing the house. Together, they put away potentially
harmful or breakable items (such as inherited china) or at least
place these things out of Ethan's reach. They don't want to put
a stop to their son's natural curiosity, but safety is important
so they also decide to put child locks on all the lower drawers
and cabinets, and to put a child gate in the kitchen doorway.

Do you have to turn your lovely home into a playground?
No, but it's better to childproof than to be constantly scolding
your kids every time they come near one of your treasures.
Again, *prevention* is key. If you're not an especially good orga-
nizer, then get help. The expression "everything in its place"
is especially useful when it comes to kids. Simple solutions,
such as having cabinets or chests where toys can be put away
at the end of the day, can really help.

SUMMARY: NURTURING YOUR CHILD'S
BRAIN DEVELOPMENT

You might want your child to graduate from Harvard Business
School and become CEO of a major international corporation

or—better yet—be able to fulfill his dreams and create a happy, productive life. There are three simple recommendations, which might not seem very remarkable, but which will help the development of every child's brain: *a quiet environment*, *being held*, and *having lots of playtime*.

A QUIET ENVIRONMENT

From the very beginning, it's good to start nurturing children's brain development. In the womb, they've known only darkness and warmth, gentle motion, and muffled sounds. Suddenly they're born into a world of bright lights and loud noises and random movement. Their sensory systems are not developed, so they can't make sense of anything yet. You can make life much easier for them by keeping them in a quiet, subdued environment in which their brain pathways can develop without being constantly shocked by overstimulation. Many cultures traditionally keep newborns in a quiet room for six full weeks before taking them outside. If it's at all possible for you to arrange this for both the new mother and the baby, it will, according to Ayurveda, allow both of them to settle into their new lives more easily.

HOLD YOUR NEWBORN

A newborn's most important sense is *touch*. Infants can only see random blobs of light and hear disconnected sounds, but research has shown that their sense of touch is quite developed. Let your newborn know that you're there, and that you love them, by *holding* them. Stroking their arms and legs also helps develop the brain's internal "body map," which plays an important role in their coordination as they learn to crawl, to walk, and to block goals.

PLAY

As children reach preschool age, don't rush them into violin and Italian lessons or create a structured play environment designed to teach them quantum physics and world geography. If you want to develop your child's maximum brain power—along with a healthy body and social skills—give him plenty of time for *unstructured* play. We can't say it any better than Regina M. Milteer and Kenneth R. Ginsburg, who discuss this in "The Importance of Play in Promoting Healthy Child Development and Maintaining Strong Parent-Child Bonds" from the American Academy of Pediatrics:

> *Play allows children to use their creativity while developing their imagination, dexterity, and physical, cognitive, and emotional strength. Play is important to healthy brain development. . . . Undirected play allows children to learn how to work in groups, to share, to negotiate, to resolve conflicts, and to learn self-advocacy skills. When play is allowed to be child driven, children practice decision-making skills, move at their own pace, discover their own areas of interest, and ultimately engage fully in the passions they wish to pursue. . . . In contrast to passive entertainment, play builds active, healthy bodies. . . . Perhaps above all, play is a simple joy that is a cherished part of childhood.*

CHAPTER 9

DHARMA PARENTING TOOLS:
The School Years,
Four to Nine

THIS IS AN EXCITING TIME when your child's imagination is unleashed as brain circuits develop further and the most mundane object can be anything he desires—a spaceship, a monster, or a castle. At this stage the child is able to think in terms of cause and effect. This is also the period when children begin to accept and value rules, which allow them to more confidently navigate life's unknowns.

YOUR CHILD'S BRAIN

Your school-age child's brain is almost as big as yours, but there's an important difference: The surface layer of the child's brain—the cortex, where all the processing takes place—*is twice as thick*. It's thicker because each neuron has twice as many connections. It is this dense brain connectivity, which allows the child to master language, learn to work in groups, and to follow rules.

Another significant brain change during this period is that two very important brain systems are now adding layers of myelin (a fatty white matter) to their output fibers. As we have mentioned, myelin insulates the neurons from interference and speeds up processing. The first part of the brain to add myelin is the motor system, which finishes around four years of age. Have you ever tried to play catch with three-year-olds? They hold their arms out. The ball hits their chest and falls on the ground, and *then* they close their arms. Because their motor neurons are not yet myelinated, it takes so long for the message to move—from eyes to brain, from brain to the spinal cord, and, finally, from the spinal cord to their arms—*that they miss the ball.* You can practice with them as long as you like, but their reactions can't speed up until the motor system has become myelinated. (Coaches of future Michael Jordans, please take note!)

The next major brain system to add myelin is the set of connections between the left and right hemispheres. This myelination begins at age seven and ends around age ten. As these connecting fibers become myelinated, information flows between the two hemispheres twenty times faster. With these faster connections, your nine-year-old can place immediate concrete experiences (processed in the left hemisphere) into a wider and more holistic context (processed in the right hemisphere). For example, a fourth grader can sort sticks according to length, a first grader cannot. The fourth grader knows that a ball of clay weighs the same when it's broken in half, while the first grader thinks it is heavier because there are more pieces.

THINKING AND LEARNING

Be alert to the amazing advances in your child's mental abilities during these years. The changes are less obvious than improved motor coordination and communication but just as dramatic. For example, if you ask your four-year-old a question, he may take a fairly long time to respond. You can almost see the question moving from the child's ears to the brain, and rumbling around in there for a while until the answer at last travels down to the child's mouth. Ask the same question to a nine-year-old and the answer will be prompt. All of this is because information travels more quickly between the hemispheres through the older child's newly myelinated connecting fibers.

As a result of this development, children can begin to understand relationships between objects. They start to grasp the concept of cause and effect and to realize that they're responsible for their actions—right or wrong. This is why children of this age look for rules and consider those rules absolute.

Logical thinking also begins to mature; they can begin to plan and reason, and are better able to express their ideas. Memory improves so they can remember details in the context of the big picture. This allows them to solve more complex problems and also to perform complex tasks that require several steps to complete. Stay attuned to your children's brain development so you can adjust your parenting skills to meet their changing needs.

APPLYING THE DHARMA PARENTING TOOLS DURING THE SCHOOL YEARS

TOOL 1: DISCOVER YOUR CHILD'S BRAIN/BODY TYPE

At this age, kids soak up rules, because rules give them control over their lives. Being rule governed, kids enjoy learning how to monitor their own brain/body type and how to address their imbalances. One of the most effective ways to determine your state of balance is through a technique of self-pulse, which is part of traditional Ayurveda. Taking your own pulse is easy to learn, and when your children are old enough you can help them follow the simple instructions in appendix 2. (You can also take courses on pulse diagnosis at mum.edu/ online.) First, master taking your own pulse, and then you can teach your children. Be sure to give them only simple instructions at first, and further details over time. Remind your children to take their pulse at different times of the day. You can make a chart for them to fill out when they detect an imbalance, and to briefly describe how they got back in balance.

TOOL 2: HEAL YOURSELF

When your child starts school, either half or full days, you'll now have time to begin to *heal yourself.* You've been reacting to emergency situations 24-7 since they were born. Now you can be proactive and start to set up a good routine for yourself. If you're working, you can luxuriate in simply dropping off and picking up your child from school, rather than having to organize child care. If you're at home in the mornings, after the kids are in school, you might set aside twenty minutes to meditate or rest. This is precious time; use it to your maximum benefit and protect it. In a couple of months, whenever your batteries feel recharged, you might want to take a class in something you enjoy. Just don't do too much too quickly, and try to do it regularly.

TOOL 3: ATTENTION AND APPRECIATION

Your attention supports and nurtures your child's development. Interests and abilities emerge at different times in every child. Your alert attention notices what ability is emerging, and your appreciation allows that ability to grow.

Supporting Your Child's Learning Style

> It's teacher conference night, and Judy and Deb are catching up on their lives as they wait to meet with their seven-year-olds' teacher. As they talk, they discover that their children are polar opposites. "Lisa is suddenly devouring books," Judy exclaims. "And yesterday she wrote a poem! It even rhymed, sort of."
>
> "What?" yelps Deb. "Jake can barely read his worksheets! I have to help him every afternoon, and he hates it!"
>
> "Maybe Ms. Moran can give you some special exercises for him," Judy says thoughtfully.
>
> Special exercises? Deb thinks, with a small surge of panic. How can he be falling behind already? He's only in second grade!

Deb doesn't need to worry about Jake's language skills being behind Lisa's—this is a normal boy-girl situation. Brain circuits develop at different rates in every child, and girls generally learn to speak much earlier than boys do. Girls also tend to use more complex sentence structures. So it's natural that Lisa is dancing across the printed page while Jake slogs along behind.

Each brain/body type has a different learning style. If Lisa is a Vata, she'll naturally be quick to learn language and be a talkative child. Language skills come easily to this type, and before you know it, they're creating their own stories and poems. Encourage these skills, but don't let your child overdo it by staying up late reading. Pitta brain/body types may also learn language skills quickly due to their intense focus and love of accomplishment.

Jake is a Kapha and will naturally, therefore, be slower learning language. This brain/body type generally takes longer to learn, but with time they will catch up and tend to retain information very well.

By thoroughly understanding how Jake's body type and brain development impact his learning style, Deb can be focused and purposeful instead of concerned. Since Jake is a Kapha, she understands that he will learn best by doing, not just by looking or listening. She can suggest that he point to each word as he reads it or even trace the letters of the words. Once the boy feels established as a reader, he'll naturally stop using these props.

The key point in helping develop your child's language skills is that *experience changes the brain*. Speak to your child in adult sentences. Read books with your son or daughter. Hearing words and sentences actually structures your child's brain and improves the ability to follow sequences of ideas.

Helping Your Child Develop Self-Control

Extensive research on young children (four to six years old) has shown that children with greater self-control grow up to be more empathetic, less fearful and angry, and better able to deal with frustration and stress. Child psychologists say that the ability to self-regulate behavior may be *the single most important predictor of success and happiness in life*. What can you do to help nurture your child's self-control?

The easiest approach is to help them repeatedly accomplish something constructive in an activity they really enjoy and which naturally excites them. It might be music or art lessons, martial arts, or team sports. A word of caution: If you push hard and your child fails, it can cost them dearly in self-confidence. So be sure your child knows that it's the fun that's important; make it clear that you don't expect a spectacular result—the Mona Lisa or a game-winning home run. Of course, you also need to be careful to choose activities that are appropriate for your son or daughter's developmental level *and* brain/body type, so the child can enjoy the activity and successfully meet the challenge.

Be careful, too, not to go overboard with structured activities. Creative play is *as important* for children at this age as it was when they were younger. For kids from four to six, a stick can be a lawn mower, a rabbit, or an invisible friend, and their pillow is a frog. The more time children spend in creative play, the more creative brain pathways are strengthened. As their brain develops, they begin to understand rules and predict the results of their actions. They can plan ahead. Creative play allows them to rehearse these new abilities. Whether they're nurturing a family of stuffed animals or organizing their friends to ambush the bad guys, unstructured child-driven play helps kids practice adult roles and develop their own ways of doing things.

NOTE FROM MOM

"BORING": THE B-WORD

In our house, using the B-word costs you twenty-five cents. We instigated this rule because we hated to hear kids whine, "Mom, I'm *bored*," and then watch their mom (or dad) scurry around to find something to keep the child entertained.

Instead, we explained that boredom comes from inside, not from outside—if you look around, there's always something interesting to see or do or think about. This encouraged their self-reliance and natural curiosity.

Not to mention that it swelled our bank account. In twenty-seven years of parenting, we've collected a grand total of seventy-five cents.

Don't Let Electronics Be a Substitute for Your Attention

Vicki takes a lasagna out of the oven and glances nervously across the room at her six-year-old son. As usual, Xander is engrossed in an electronic game, and as usual, Vicki feels a pang of concern, along with some guilt.

Vicki is a single mom who relies heavily on TV and electronic games to keep her son occupied while she is busy with household chores. Xander certainly appears to be happy, healthy, and smart for his age, but shouldn't he be running around more and playing outside? Vicki also wonders how much time in front of a screen is healthy for a child.

At lunch the next day, she confides her concerns to her coworker Bruce, a dad who has two children around Xander's age. Bruce is sympathetic. "It's tough being a single parent," he says. "My sister is a single mom, and sometimes she gets so tired she can't see the obvious solution.

"I have a question for you: why are you cooking and cleaning by yourself while Xander is playing computer games by himself?"

It takes Vicki a minute to realize how brilliant yet how obvious Bruce's perception is. "Wow! We could work together, it would be fun for both of us, and he'd be off his electronics."

On the way to school the next morning, Vicki asks her son if he'd like pizza for dinner that night. When the boy stops cheering, she adds, "But I need your help making it. I'll show you how to do everything."

Xander is enthusiastic in the kitchen that evening, grating cheese, opening a can of tomato sauce, and spreading the cheese on top of the pizza. He even agrees that people who cook should also help clean. He and his mom sing silly songs while they wash the dishes and wipe down the counters.

The next weekend, Vicki expands her strategy by suggesting that if they both clean the house on Saturday morning, they'll have time for a fun excursion in the afternoon.

Xander certainly doesn't abandon his computer games completely, but Vicki feels that his use of time is becoming much more balanced and also better for their relationship.

Vicki's parenting strategy is helping her son's development in two very important ways:

First, the boy is spending lots of time helping his mom, and he's learning much more than just how to make pizza or a bed—he's learning social skills and how to follow instructions. He's also experiencing the fulfillment of completing a task. Research has shown that the children who do best at school followed their parents around when they were young and helped with daily activities as they grew older. For example, while mom cooked, they had their own bread dough and rolling pin. These children become more curious and more open to new experiences; they deal with conflict better and are happier. Children who do poorly in school have been shown to be those who were put into playpens in their first years or set in front of the TV at school age. A child in a playpen doesn't have a chance to explore the world or experience the good feeling from completing a challenging task.

Second, Xander is spending less time with his electronics. In the past he wasn't comfortable making friends, but now that he's spending more time talking with his mom, he's figuring out how to talk to other kids as well. He's getting more exercise too, because some of those special Saturday excursions include games of Frisbee, biking, and running through the park. Vicki is going to encourage him to join a T-ball team in the spring.

But what if you try something like this and your kids don't want to cooperate? You ask if they want pizza for dinner and they mumble, "I don't care what we eat." You suggest an excursion and they say they'd rather stay home. If this is what's happening, there are two areas you must address: If you feel it's important to decrease their screen time, then you'll have to find a way to do it, either by getting them to cooperate or by setting limits in spite of their protests. More important, you need to address the underlying cause of their noncooperation, which is likely to be *an imbalance in their physiology.*

Imbalances arise in all brain/body types: Too much Kapha can cause stubbornness—a mulish refusal to allow any change—and possessiveness, so Kaphas might feel their world will end if you take away their gaming device. Aggravated Pittas love the focus of electronic games and Internet surfing, and they can rise up in anger if they feel their electronic rights are being thwarted. Restless Vatas may find that the fast pace and frenetic graphics of a computer game are the only things that can capture their attention and keep them focused; these Vatas may feel lost without the constant presence and stimulation of their electronic buddies. In every case, put attention on restoring your child's balance through a careful choice of diet and activities.

But that's a long-term solution; what about right now? You could start with a variation of Vicki's strategy. Figure out an irresistible treat and tell them you need their help so that you'll have time to take them to the ice rink or the lake or the new aquarium. Or help them to get them started on a new *nonelectronic* hobby. With younger children, you may need to adopt that same hobby yourself. For example, if your child shows an interest in cars or motorcycles, buy a model kit and work on it together. "Hey, Erik, I bought this model Ferrari but I'm not sure I can put it together. Can you help me figure it out?" Expect the process to take time and attention, especially when you first start to implement changes.

NOTE FROM MOM

CONTROL THOSE ELECTRONICS

Before you start worrying about your children's screen time, do a quick reality check: How are they doing in school? Do they have healthy friendships, in person and online? Do they seem well integrated at home, participating in family chores and excursions? If all your answers are yes, then their electronics use doesn't seem to be doing much harm.

If you decide they should cut down on their electronics, how do you it? There's software you can use to limit their total online time each day and control what hours they can log on. Your cell phone provider allows you to limit their talk time, texting, and data usage. You can also turn off the household Wi-Fi well before bedtime.

But some psychologists now recommend that you don't focus on limiting electronics use to a specific total per day. Instead, create "electronics-free zones": no phones or handhelds in the car, no electronics at meals or on family fun nights. Computers are okay for homework, but no other devices. And no electronics in the bedrooms at night—all those wonderful devices spend the night together at the recharging station.

It's best to start this as soon as your child is old enough to have his own phone, game box, or computer. Internet addiction can begin in the early school years and flower into full toxicity in the teen years. It's much easier to set limits at the beginning than to add restrictions later on. Still, better later than never!

TOOL 4: ROUTINES

Children from four to nine years old love rules—psychologists call it "rule-governed behavior." As the connecting fibers start to develop their layers of myelin and speed up communication between the left and right hemispheres of the brain, children begin to understand their immediate concrete experiences in a wider, more holistic context. They begin to see the patterns in their life: this is what I do on school days, this is what our family does on weekends, and this is what happens when a friend comes over to play. What used to seem random now begins to make sense, and children embrace the rules and routines that create the structure they can use to order their life.

Going to School

The biggest change in children's daily routine during these years is school. Think of the immense change it makes in their lives: at age four their day is preschool, playdates, and family time. By age nine, school dominates their waking hours, and adults praise them for getting good grades or winning a spelling bee.

Children are naturally nervous about their first day of school: What will it be like? Will my teacher be nice? Will the other kids like me? What if I don't know what to do? Here are some steps you can take to decrease their anxiety:

- Check with the school: many schools let you bring your child to see the building, visit their new classroom, and meet their teacher before school starts; some have official "meet your teacher" days.

- Rehearse going to school: familiarize your child with their new school routine ahead of time. Pretend it's a school day and have your son or daughter get up on time, get dressed, and eat breakfast. Then walk or drive the child to school, pointing out landmarks so he knows the route. Show your child which door to use, and if possible how to find the classroom. Don't forget about lunch—either bring a lunch from home or rehearse what to do in the cafeteria. And be sure your child knows what to do when the final bell rings: where to meet you and how to get there. Practice the whole routine two or three times before that important first day.
- Find them a buddy: the first day of school is much easier with a friend, so try to arrange a couple of summer playdates with other kids who'll be in the same class.

Remember that it's not just first graders who feel nervous about the first day of school. Every year, even up to high school, it's a good idea to take your child to meet the new teacher and find the new classroom or homeroom.

Family Chores

This is an ideal age to introduce regular chores as part of the family routine. Have a family meeting, formal or informal, to decide what needs to be done each day and each week, and to figure out who will be responsible for what. Of course, chores should be age appropriate. But if your ambitious eight-year-old wants to take on a chore that you think is too much for him—mowing the lawn, for example—let him be responsible for it, but also let him know he'll be getting lots of help. A child obviously can't run the power lawn mower, but he can be in charge of reminding Dad or big sister that it's time to mow, and making sure they don't miss any corners. They can certainly pull out that pesky crabgrass along the walk and help clean up the mower and push it back into the garage.

Once chores are assigned, allow some time for the kids to learn how to do each job properly. Maybe they can start by doing the chore with you or with a trustworthy older sibling. Have them help you make a "chore chart" for the bulletin board or refrigerator. Stickers are good rewards when younger children have completed their chores and checked off all the boxes; older ones will probably prefer some extra computer time.

NOTE FROM MOM

HELICOPTER PARENTING

Resist the urge to become a "helicopter parent," hovering over your kids to make sure they're occupied with useful/creative activities, or that their teachers understand them, or that they're finishing their homework rather than surfing the Net, etc. Children need to learn *self*-discipline and *self*-motivation. If you want them to be successful and happy, let them find their own voice, do their own thing, and march to the beat of their own drummer.

To cure yourself of helicopter tendencies, check out Alexander McCall Smith's 44 Scotland Street novels. Irene Pollock, mother of precocious six-year-old Bertie, is an excellent example of how *not* to parent.

One simple chore is everyone tidying and cleaning their own bedroom. Do not, however, impose your sense of cleanliness on them. If your children are young, begin simply: just sit in the middle of the room and ask where they think each toy should go. Children can also help put away clean laundry and make their beds. Some parents have a specific time each day—around dinnertime or at the beginning of the bedtime routine—when they take a quick look at each child's bedroom and ask the child to put away at least some of the things that are strewn around.

TOOL 5: MANAGE MELTDOWNS

Good news: Meltdowns are at a minimum during these years. Your child is finished with the terrible twos and hasn't yet reached adolescence. And if he does have a meltdown, it's generally easier to handle for both of you. Before this, you mostly gave your preschooler nonverbal support, with a few soothing words to help calm him down. Continue with this nonverbal support—holding your child and rubbing his back—but also spend more time talking together.

At this age, children can understand and will profit from time-outs. The recommended time period for a time-out is *one minute for each year of the child's age.* Your children's language and reasoning skills are growing, so once they've calmed down you can reason with them. At this age, kids have sufficient cognitive development to understand when they've done something wrong and to think about it. Once the meltdown is over, it's important to discuss what happened, and give your child time to reflect on what happened—but *without guilt*—so that she can internalize the lesson. Take your cue from your child's attitude at this point; if she has already learned the lesson, you don't need to belabor the point. Your child will simply stop listening if you do, so keep it as short and as calm as possible.

TOOL 6: ANTICIPATE AND ADAPT

For your first three years of parenting, you may have been scrambling to keep up with all the parenting chores. From ages four to nine, things calm down because your child's exuberant brain development has reached its peak level, supporting the steady growth of reasoning ability, memory, planning, and a sense of responsibility.

During these years, children are adapting to the increasing expectations of the adults in their lives. Everyone used to coo at them no matter what they did—"Oh, isn't she cute!"—but now they're expected to "behave," and adults frown at them for acting like three-year-olds.

Anticipate these increased expectations in a very practical way of teaching your children manners. This is a great time to start, because you can take advantage of the rule-based behavior that dominates this age. Your child has already been learning table manners, of course, at every meal you eat together. Mostly children learn by example, but now they're old enough for you to start reinforcing examples by explaining what good manners are. It's easy to gently remind them if they forget to ask politely or to say "thank you" when someone passes them the butter. Make sure they ask to be excused before leaving the table. When you walk into a building, step back so your child can hold the door for you (if it's not too heavy)—this is how he will learn to provide the same courtesy for any adult. If you're riding the bus together, offer your seat to an older person or a pregnant woman, and explain the principle to your child. The next time, prompt them to offer their own seat.

Manners are important, but even more important is the innate consideration of others that underlies good manners. For example, if you are giving your dinner partner your full attention and are sincerely interested in them, it doesn't matter very much if you knock over the salt or use the wrong fork. Your children learn true respect for others by experiencing it themselves—which brings us back to the value of attention and appreciation as a parenting tool. Your child models his behavior after yours, not just on the superficial level of good manners, but also on the more profound level of treating other people as important and worthy human beings.

NOTE FROM MOM

THE MANNERS GAME

Our oldest daughter started learning manners from her grandma even before she was out of her high chair. Grandma taught her to take "lady bites" and pat her lips with her napkin. It was fun for both of them, a game they shared that taught an important skill.

Some families use this "game" approach to upgrade everyone's manners: Once a month or so, they set aside a weekend family night to role-play and practice correct table manners. They'll have a formal dinner with candlelight, all the possible plates and silverware, and top-level manners. You might want to practice like this a week before Thanksgiving or any large gathering. You can also practice introductions, making a game out of tricky precedence questions: "Grandma, I'd like you to meet the king of Jordan—or should I say, 'Your Majesty, I'd like you to meet my grandmother'? Which takes precedence: age, gender, or royalty?" It's unlikely that most of us will ever be confronted by such a question, but it's good for the whole family to learn the basics of everyday manners.

It can be fun to check out a book of manners from the library and read the minutely detailed instructions about social niceties. One book, for example, explained that a gentleman always removes his glove when shaking hands; a lady need not remove her glove, but she should say, "Pardon my glove." This has become a byword in our family anytime we make an etiquette error: "Oh, my dear, pardon my glove!"

Take time during these more predictable years to anticipate what your child will need to create a stable foundation for the vast brain and hormone changes coming up in adolescence. Start building the foundation now through responsibilities at home, which build children's self-reliance and self-confidence. Support their interest in extracurricular activities, which give them the satisfaction of accomplishment, as well as by letting them know, by your attention and appreciation, that you respect and cherish them.

DEVELOPING YOUR PARENTING STYLE

"Okay, Dylan. Now it's really time to get off the Game Boy," Jenny says to her seven-year-old. "It's waaay past your bedtime."

"No," the boy replies sullenly.

"Come on! I mean it. You're going to be exhausted tomorrow."

"Shut up!" shouts Dylan. "You can't tell me what to do! You're a dumbhead!" Jenny can see that he's beginning to go into one of his rages; as usual, she doesn't know what to do.

Dylan has always been a demanding child, but

Jenny and her husband, Nick, found him so adorable that they could never bear to discipline him properly.

A few days ago, however, the school principal called to say that he had hit another child on the playground. Dylan is big for his age and is showing signs of becoming a bully. Nick and Jenny are both wondering what they are doing wrong.

Jenny and Nick have created this problem by an overly permissive style of parenting, high on warmth but low on accountability. The warmth is great, but Dylan needs to start experiencing the consequences of his behavior. His parents haven't given him any feedback about his outbursts, which seem to be escalating into antisocial behavior—but his classmates and teachers certainly will. And Dylan's going to find it very hard to make friends if he keeps hitting them. The problem is that he hasn't learned any other way to behave. Research reports that children with permissive parents tend to become increasingly aggressive as they get older, and as teenagers have nearly triple the rate of heavy drinking. You're doing your child a big favor when you teach him how to behave within boundaries. At first, you set the boundaries, and when children get older, they can participate in setting them. By the time they move out on their own, they'll need to be completely self-reliant and self-regulating, because you won't be around to do it for them.

Some parents would strongly suggest that Jenny and Nick capture Dylan's attention by yelling at him, and that a good spanking would be an effective form of punishment when the boy hits someone else. This, however, would be both a mistake and a myopic short-term solution. As we said before, *How can we ask our children to stop hitting and hurting others when we are hitting and hurting them?* Authoritarian parenting tries to teach good behavior by punishing children when they step outside their parents' notion of boundaries. This "boot camp" type of parent believes that parents are the authority—they're older and more experienced, and they know what's best for their kids. They're in charge—and their children will be better off if they just do what they're told. These parents don't explain or discuss, but they're good at belittling and punishing. Children of authoritarian parents are usually quite well behaved, but their self-esteem is low, they're less resourceful, and they often have poor social skills, including long-term intimacy problems. They also tend to rebel when they become teenagers. Since their parents have set themselves up as the ultimate authority, these kids don't have a chance to learn how to set boundaries for themselves. What will happen when they grow up?

Authoritative, in contrast to authoritarian, parenting involves setting clear boundaries and rules while responding to your child's individual needs. Authoritative parents create a nurturing environment in which children are treated fairly and respectfully, family policies and decisions are discussed, and everyone feels comfortable questioning the rules and making mistakes.

Your parenting style—the way you teach and discipline your child—*is vital for the creation of self-regulating pathways* in your child's brain. Our kids imitate both our good and our bad behavior, and both styles of action lead to the strengthening of specific neural pathways that become the basis for future behavior—good, bad, or indifferent. *With positive and effective parenting,* your children will become more independent and self-confident, and develop a sense of right and wrong that will help them resist negative peer pressure.

NOTE FROM MOM

SCAFFOLDING

"Scaffolding" is a simple educational concept: provide support so that your child can master a demanding task with your help, and then gradually withdraw that support until they can stand on their own. As a parent and a coach, be alert to give just enough scaffolding so your child can succeed. You're not "babying them along"—you're providing the support they need to get started. Be careful not to take over their project; just bring out different ways to approach it.

Scaffolding is different for every age—a toddler trying to solve a puzzle or a teen writing an essay for a college application. In each case, you're supporting your child's activities, but you're not telling him what to do—and certainly not doing it for him. You're functioning as your child's not-yet-developed frontal lobes, providing a hands-on example of how to plan and reason.

CHAPTER 10

DHARMA PARENTING TOOLS: The Preteen and Teenage Years, Ten to Seventeen

A TEN-YEAR-OLD ENJOYS RULES AND GUIDELINES, and loves to spend time with you, either working or playing. But fasten your seat belt because seventeen-year-olds *know* that no rule is absolute. Rules are different in different contexts, and teens *love* to test boundaries. Then there's the fact that most teenagers prefer to be with their peers—rather than their loving family. And all of these changes are driven by changes in your child's brain.

PRETEEN AND TEEN BRAIN DEVELOPMENT

From the ages of three to ten, your child has more connections between brain circuits than at any other time of life. From ages ten to seventeen, they lose 1 to 2 percent of these brain connections each year, in a process called "pruning." Pruning follows the principle of "use it or lose it." Connections that are being used remain, while those that are not are absorbed back into the neuron. This process is similar to pruning a shrub or tree. When we trim away spindly branches and shoots, the plant grows thicker, and fruit and leaves become more abundant. In our brain, pruning ensures that limited cortical resources are devoted to increasing those brain connections that are currently being used. This results in a brain with neural pathways tailor-made to meet its owner's needs.

Not only are your child's brain connections being sculpted by the pruning process, but the *nature* of those connections is also changing. Remember myelin? It's that fatty substance, or white matter, which *insulates* neural connections from interference and *speeds up* processing. Between birth and age four, your child's motor system was myelinating; from age seven to ten, right/left hemisphere connections were myelinating. Now it's time for the prefrontal cortex (the front of the brain, directly over the eyes) and all of its connections to begin maturing. This starts around age eleven or twelve in girls, a couple years later in boys, and continues through to age twenty-five.

How does all of this affect your adolescent? Circuits in the back of your child's brain create a picture of what's happening right now. Like film images on a screen, each new experience replaces the earlier image. It's as if we're watching a real time "movie" of our life. Images are then sent to the front of the brain—the prefrontal cortex—which is the brain's "CEO" or boss. The prefrontal cortex places the concrete present—what's happening right now—into the larger context of past and future experience, plans, goals, and values. Myelin around prefrontal brain connections increases the speed of processing, and this optimizes communication between different brain areas. *The addition of myelin to this area allows the more holistic and mature perspective of the frontal executive areas to influence our perception and decision making.*

Before the prefrontal areas are myelinated, a teenager might write a very sincere essay about the dangers of drinking one day, and then get drunk the following weekend. Before myelination, commands from the prefrontal areas move more slowly along neural pathways than the sensory images flooding the back of the brain. When the teenager was writing that essay, he had plenty of time to think about the subject, so it didn't matter that his prefrontal areas worked more slowly. But when he's out with friends, and must make quick decisions, the reasoning and "bigger picture" (from the frontal lobes) are overcome by the excitement of the moment. Passionate emotions drive a teenager's decisions. In adults the line of communication between the prefrontal cortex and the rest of the brain is well established. If the adult prefrontal area could speak to the emotional part of the teenage brain, it might say, "Don't drink and drive. It's not safe!" But the conversation would be very different for the teenager, whose prefrontal cortex is not yet completely developed: "It's no big deal to drink and drive! This is fun! I can take that next corner at seventy-five miles an hour, *easy.*"

As the parent of a teenager, you must act as their prefrontal cortex. This doesn't mean being a helicopter parent, checking every move your teen makes to be sure they're safe and making good decisions. Rather, it means that you help them prepare for any tricky situation that might arise. For example, when your teenage son or daughter is going to a party, make sure that they understand and commit to the concept of a designated driver. If the roads are icy, don't just say "be careful" when you hand them the car keys. Instead, remind them of the specific driving techniques they may need: "If you start to skid, what do you do?" "How fast can you take that sharp curve by Jody's house when it's this icy?" This primes the teenager's frontal areas before they leave, so there's a greater chance that *messages from the prefrontal cortex will be heard.*

NOTE FROM MOM

TO PARENTS OF GIRLS

The brains of adolescent boys develop two or three years later than girls' brains do. Make sure that your daughter knows this: If a boy suggests something that seems risky or dangerous—or that she just doesn't want to do—she should remember that his brain is back where hers was three years ago. She's the one (maybe the only one) who can foresee consequences and use her common sense to judge impulsive decisions.

THINKING AND LEARNING

Neural pruning dominates the young teenager's experience. The brain circuits change every day as less frequently used connections drop off. This affects their ability to focus and reason because they can't rely on their brains to function the way they did last week, or even yesterday. This also means that the teen's sense of self is constantly in flux. It's no exaggeration to say that the brain that kids this age wake up with is not the same brain they went to sleep with!

As frontal executive areas mature, the adolescent's individuality emerges. When they were younger, they could only think about concrete objects: "How can I make my remote control car go faster?" "Can I sleep with my head at the other end of my bed?"

Now they can think about thinking—about ideas and concepts: "Why do I need to go to bed before midnight?" "Would I like to be vegetarian?" Teenagers need to discover their own thoughts and values; it's part of their mental development. They need to question *everything*, and they will come up with elaborate arguments to defend their new ways of seeing the world—at least until the next day, when they have a completely different worldview.

Rules provide tools to organize life's variety and challenges. As the brain continues to mature, however, teenagers increasingly begin to realize that rules are context dependent. What used to be black and white now has many shades of gray, or maybe Technicolor. Remember this the next time your teenage daughter asks why she has to clean her room—after all, it's *her* room. And why does she have to be in bed by ten on a school night? She can handle being tired in the morning! This is all part of a natural coming-of-age process, and your response is crucial.

The ability to question assumptions is valuable throughout life, and it's very important that you support your teenager's newfound autonomy while providing clear boundaries. Whatever you do, never try to win an argument with your teen. They will always manage to have the last word. Work *with* your teen to explore his perspective.

Don't take your teens' overly emphatic comments too seriously. By this we mean listen and reflect on what they're saying but don't let their statements provoke you or hurt you. If they remark passionately, "Money isn't important," don't get angry because you've been working overtime to save for their college tuition. They're simply exercising their growing ability to adopt a point of view; next week they may have an entirely different one. Think *with* them. And bring up the consequences of their statements. Ask if they think money is useful sometimes—for instance, to pay their cell phone bill. Engage them as they explore and test possibilities.

APPLYING DHARMA PARENTING TOOLS DURING THE PRETEEN AND TEENAGE YEARS

TOOL 1: DISCOVER YOUR CHILD'S BRAIN/BODY TYPE

Understanding your teenager's brain/body type gives you a distinct advantage in the inevitable coming-of-age clashes with your teenager. And there are three sources of behavior you need to consider. First, your teen's body type may be out of balance due to the weather, food, or various stressors. Second, the depth of his thinking and actions will reflect the constant reorganization of the brain, such as the pruning of connections and maturation of circuits in the prefrontal executive areas. Third, puberty naturally involves wide emotional swings—your teen really has no idea what's going on as they ride an emotional roller coaster of hormones.

From age ten to seventeen, brain and hormonal changes contribute more to your teenager's behavior than body type does. However, keep all three in mind—body type, brain changes, and puberty—as you try to help your son or daughter move through this phase of life.

> *"Go ahead! Take my stuff and wreck it!"* Karen cries, anger competing with self-pity for the upper hand. *"Take it all, why don't you, and just leave me a few broken paintbrushes."*

"Oh, don't give me that garbage!" her younger sister, Megan, shoots back. "I just borrowed a few brushes and didn't clean them right away. Stop taking everything so personally. Here!" She throws the brushes at Karen, and Karen screams.
"You big baby!" Megan yells. "Grow up!"

Will and Joan's two daughters are having entirely different experiences as they go through puberty. Karen has always been a somewhat delicate and artistic child; now she's become highly emotional, with a tendency to internalize her feelings—especially before her period. Karen often sees herself as a victim and, in extreme situations, she can become self-destructive.

Her sister, Megan, was a strong athlete and a focused student as a child, and has become more bossy and temperamental as she goes through puberty, to the point of being physically aggressive toward her older sister. This, unfortunately, feeds into Karen's victim psychology. Their parents have their hands full, trying to ease both their girls through this rough patch and at the same time help them figure out who on earth they are.

For girls, the onset of puberty occurs around age ten or eleven and, as they become teenagers, is accompanied by dramatic physical and emotional changes. Puberty tends to exaggerate otherwise manageable latent tendencies in all brain/body types. Puberty floods a girl's body with estrogen, and estrogen increases emotional sensitivity. And not only is she undergoing hormonal changes, but her brain is going through its last major transformation. We can see this in both Karen and Megan: they're trying to figure out who they are, and the process isn't easy because their brains *and* their bodies are in a state of flux. Brain circuits, which once provided a stable picture of the world and supported balanced inner emotions, now generate wildly changing thoughts and strong emotions.

Will and Joan's oldest daughter, Karen, is a typical Vata with a wide range of emotional swings, from high excitement to low depression. Karen is constantly "trying on" various feelings and questioning and doubting herself. These tendencies can be found to some degree in each of the brain/body types during puberty. When Vata girls are in good balance, however, they can be remarkably imaginative and flexible.

The younger daughter, Megan, is a typical Pitta whose emotional upheavals come out as rage rather than tears. When imbalanced, these types may be bossy, impatient, irritable, and angry. It's as if they have a switch inside that turns their emotional pilot light to high at a moment's notice. The trigger may be as simple as not eating on time, being overheated, or eating spicy foods. And once they're inflamed, you can't talk with them because they can't hear reason; they can only feel their inner fire. Their intense feelings often come out as negative statements that cut others deeply. When they're in good balance, however, Pitta girls are full of passion, organization, and drive. No problem is too big. They seek challenges and love to test themselves. And adversity is seen as a chance to overcome a challenge.

Teen girls with the Kapha brain/body type tend to be more stable than their Vata or Pitta friends. But if they are out of balance, they can become withdrawn, selfish, or depressed. Kapha has the quality of heaviness, so it may be difficult to get your Kapha teen moving, not just in the morning, but whenever life feels overwhelming to them. Kapha brain/body types are generally compassionate and like to help others, so you can motivate them by saying that you need their help—even if the only thing you need help with is getting them out of bed.

About all you really can do for your daughter during this period is to help her *stay in balance*, whatever kind of brain/body type she has. Help her maintain a reasonable schedule in the midst of all the activities and socializing, so she gets enough rest and nutrition. You also need to be an immovable, utterly reliable touchstone as she undergoes these tremendous changes, and not be swayed by her storms—even when they're directed toward you. By understanding what's going on in your daughter's brain and body, you can keep a calm perspective so she knows she can count on your love and support.

> *Basketball practice has officially started, and Coach Johnston is talking to the team at the side of the court, going over the schedule for the next couple of weeks. Hearing footsteps, the coach looks up, just in time to see Austin take a running leap and land on the scorekeeper's table next to them. The table collapses.*
>
> *"Austin," Coach exclaims, "you broke the table!"*
>
> *Austin picks himself up, looking slightly dazed, and says, "Coach, the table isn't broken. It's fine."*

This actually happened; we heard it from the coach himself. Let's look at the situation from Austin's viewpoint:

> *When Austin goes to his locker after school, he finds Mia at her locker a few feet away. Mia smiles at him and asks about their English assignment, and the boy is so overwhelmed he can hardly come up with a coherent reply. She's so cute, so smart, so nice. . . .*
>
> *Now that he finally has his license (third try), maybe he can ask her out, maybe even to the winter formal. Mia walks down the stairs and out the front*

*door with him. After watching her wave good-bye
and turn away, he suddenly realizes that he's really,
really late for basketball practice. This means ten laps,
at least. Austin takes off, running, for the gym.*

*Sure enough, Coach Johnston is already talking to
the team. Desperate, Austin thinks he can join them
faster if he jumps over the table instead of walking
around it—but his spectacular leap falls short and he
crashes. He knows that he's created a scene and
wrecked the table, but he wants to reassure Coach
that he's not hurt. He's so worried about the table,
though, that the words come out all wrong, and he
says, "Coach, the table isn't broken. It's fine."*

Like Megan and Karen, Austin has been hit by the double
whammy of puberty and brain changes. The steep rise in
boys' testosterone levels at the onset of puberty gives them
higher mental and physical energy, greater work capacity, increased strength, increased muscle mass, and more aggressive
behavior. Psychologically, testosterone leads to improved confidence (and overconfidence), motivation, and concentration.
It also causes a decrease in sensory acuity. Couple these hormonal changes with the still slow connection between the
brain's executive center and its emotional center, and it's a
wonder that any boys (or their parents) survive the teenage
years.

Elevated levels of testosterone also fuel aggression and increase risk taking. If your teenage son is a Pitta brain/body
type, he *thrives* on competition—and with the onset of puberty, his tendency to dominate may become risky or even
violent. A good outlet for his almost boundless energy and
need to control is organized sports, which teach him to play

by the rules, work with a team, and stick to a schedule. If your Pitta teen isn't the athletic type, help him find another organized activity that will fulfill his need to excel: science fair, theater, or music.

Teenage boys who are Vata brain/body types are also thrill seekers, but they tend to seek emotional and artistic challenges. Do everything you can to keep your Vata teen rested and on a good schedule.

Teenage boys who are Kapha brain/body types are the most grounded physically and emotionally—even when going through puberty. When they're out of balance, however, they still need your attention to help them keep moving and challenged.

TOOL 2: HEAL YOURSELF

Teens are exploring the limits of their physical and mental abilities. At the same time, they're testing the limits of your patience, understanding, and creativity. Then there's the increasingly demanding schedule of extracurricular activities: chauffeuring teenagers to practice, chaperoning activities, and attending performances. You need to be in top form physically and mentally so that you have enough mental and emotional energy to properly parent your teen. *Make sure you are getting enough rest,* and be proactive in changing your lifestyle to support your well-being. Do you want to change your diet, learn to meditate, join an exercise class? See if you can get your teen involved too—he might enjoy exploring these possibilities with you.

TOOL 3: ATTENTION AND APPRECIATION

Adolescents are experimenting with adult lifestyle choices, and your willing ear provides a supportive sounding board for their new ideas. Be genuinely interested as they explore different cultures, ideas, and ways of looking at the world. Ask them questions about the consequences of different choices. Exploring issues will help to structure reflective thinking in your teen as his prefrontal executive brain circuits are developing.

> *Everyone is quiet on the drive home from the meeting with Ben's high school principal. His parents, Jack and Lori, are at a loss for words, and Ben is both silent and remote.*
>
> *He's always been a great kid. He took guitar lessons and played on the soccer team until he was fifteen. With high grades in most of his classes, he planned to go to college.*
>
> *But in his junior year, Ben started smoking marijuana, jamming late into the night with his new band. Six months later he was using pot regularly. Then, on his seventeenth birthday, Ben was caught smoking marijuana in a washroom at his school and was suspended. Even worse, it seems to Jack and Lori that he doesn't really care.*

This is the time for Ben's parents to make up for their past lack of attention. They should have taken turns staying up late and welcoming him home at curfew time. Then they would have noticed the smell of marijuana and the change in his behavior when he was fifteen.

At this point, they need to encourage Ben to talk. The marijuana law is confusing for teens. Adults who are twenty-one and older are allowed to buy an ounce of marijuana in some states, so Ben is wondering why he should be suspended.

Rather than having a hypothetical conversation about the legalities of marijuana, Jack and Lori could ask their son what he would like to do during his suspension. Have him suggest possible actions. Some will be imposed on him by the school—seeing a counselor monthly. Others Ben can suggest—community service to help other teens who are using drugs, or finding musicians who don't need drugs to feel they're being creative.

Once Ben begins to open up, they could ask how he feels when he smokes marijuana, and whether he knows how marijuana affects the brain. Well-designed research has reported that marijuana use slows down activity in the prefrontal executive circuits, the memory system, and the motor system. Chronic marijuana use, especially when started in the teen years, leads to chronic effects on prefrontal circuits, resulting in difficulties in planning and grasping the big picture.

It's vital for Ben's parents to include him in creating rules and consequences. If he's involved in the discussion, he's far more likely to comply with the consequences. For example, one of the consequences could be a strict curfew, which can become more lenient as he alters his behavior. If Ben is late and misses his curfew, it's important that his parents refrain from argument or criticism. Instead, they should simply tell him that he needs to come home fifteen minutes earlier—and it's nonnegotiable. It's their job as parents to *work with Ben* so he can meet his curfew and conform to any other consequences.

> *"You guys shouldn't get to tell me what I can wear!*
> *You don't know anything about fashion!" Brynn yells.*

Her mom, Jan, snorts, "Well, we certainly know that we can't afford to buy, buy, buy all day long!"

Brynn has three more years of high school, and her parents are already exhausted with ongoing battles over her wardrobe. Since she became a teenager, Brynn only wants to wear expensive designer clothes and revealing outfits that shock both her parents. One of Brynn's arguments is that "all the important people"—meaning movie stars and rock musicians—wear tight-fitting and revealing clothing from top designers.

Jan decides to divide and conquer, putting attention on one problem at a time. The first issue is the cost of clothes. This is fairly straightforward: The amount spent on clothing is necessarily limited by the family's budget. Jan and Brynn could sit and calculate a clothing allowance, which Brynn can then augment by babysitting on weekends if she wishes.

It doesn't take very long before Brynn decides to buy an accessory or two with a high-fashion label, which decimates her budget. At this point, Jan can help her daughter learn to stretch her budget by taking her to sales and discount stores.

The second issue is more complex: What is the effect of wearing provocative clothes? Billions of dollars are spent on advertising to influence Brynn to spend as much money as possible on makeup and clothing, and the media's focus on celebrities wearing tight, revealing outfits is inescapable. Jan needs to explain to Brynn that wearing skimpy clothes sends a very real signal to males, which *turns off* the thinking centers in their brains—and *turns on* their arousal centers. Some young girls are coaxed into viewing provocative clothing as a celebration of the female figure. But the reality is that revealing clothing turns guys on. They won't be concerned with who she is, what she thinks, or how she feels.

As the next step, Jan could start looking at fashion magazines with Brynn and ask what Brynn thinks would look best on her. If she enthuses over a completely inappropriate outfit, Jan could point to a less skimpy one and say, "I think this color blue would look fabulous on you," or "This style would make you look taller." The following weekend, they might turn their shopping excursion into a mutual "help me figure out what to wear"—Jan could ask Brynn for advice on a new suit to wear to work.

Resolving this delicate situation requires a lot of attention on Jan's part but it could pay off in an unexpected way: Because she's careful to always appreciate Brynn's opinion and choices, rather than belittle or criticize them, Jan is becoming better friends with her daughter. Brynn might even begin to ask her mom for advice about nonfashion issues.

TOOL 4: ROUTINES

Teenagers behave as if they want complete freedom—but what they *need* are rules and routines. And they'll constantly push boundaries to see how "real" the rules are. Prepare yourself for this onslaught by carefully considering (*before* you're challenged) which routines and rules are absolute and which can be negotiated. It's best if there can be some give-and-take, so be creative and give yourself and your teenager room to negotiate.

As preteens become teenagers, their schoolwork becomes more demanding and they may participate in more after-school activities. Sit down together and figure out exactly when they'll have time in their schedule for chores, homework, exercise, socializing, and—since yes, they do have to eat and to rest—for meals and sleep. If they want to add just one more activity, ask them to show you exactly where it will fit in.

As parents, we always want to know what we can do to nurture our child's brain development. *The best thing we can do for teens is make sure they get enough sleep.* The massive changes the teenage brain is going through use up so many resources that these kids need even more sleep than they did a few years ago. If they don't get at least eight to nine hours of sleep a night, their very important executive centers simply won't be able to develop as quickly or as profoundly.

Bedtime and curfew can become a difficult issue as your teen gets older. Work together to set the rules, and they'll be more likely to accept them without constant argument. You might create a system so they can "earn" a little later curfew on weekends if they finish their chores, get top grades, or get to bed on time the rest of the week. And rather than command them to be home on time, try asking them as they leave, "What time will you be home?" Then you can say: "Great." (At this point there may be some attempt to renegotiate.) "If something happens and you'll be late, be sure to give us a call." Always wait up for them, with a hug and some welcoming comment like, "How did it go? Sleep well. See you in the morning." It's all part of our job.

The second major consideration for raising teens is regular exercise. Exercise increases blood flow to the brain. Higher blood flow brings more nutrients to the brain. Thus adequate exercise is essential to support the major brain transformations that characterize the teen years.

NOTE FROM MOM

STRENGTH IN NUMBERS

When our oldest girl was in sixth grade, we had a parent meeting and set up guidelines for curfew and social functions. For example, no basketball games on school nights, and parties had to end by 10:00 p.m. Every year we updated: as freshmen they could stay through halftime on school nights; parties ended by 11:00 p.m.; also, no single dating.

This completely eliminated the argument "But all my friends are doing it!" Setting boundaries—and maintaining them—can be quite a challenge, especially with teenagers. It's great to have a team of parents as your understanding and supportive buddies.

TOOL 5: MANAGE MELTDOWNS

Teenagers are going through enormous physiological transformations—neural pruning, myelinating prefrontal circuits, surging hormones, changing social roles, and changing expectations. Your teenager doesn't know who he is a lot of the time, and you don't know whether today you're dealing with the reasonable version of your child or the temperamental version.

As long as no one's getting hurt, don't hold this against them. Give your teenagers space to deal with their internal turmoil, allow them to change their moods, and above all, *keep the lines of communication open.* Use your intuition to check whether they need to talk it through with you, be by themselves to settle down, or just be near you while they gather themselves together.

TOOL 6: ANTICIPATE AND ADAPT

We don't need to say much about adapting to the parents of toddlers or teenagers. And if you've survived to the teen years, you're very familiar with, if not a master of, this tool. The teenage years are not only an explosive period of growth for your child—you're growing too! Like it or not, your basic convictions are being questioned. On the plus side, this can clarify your thinking and make your outlook more flexible so you're better able to see other people's points of view.

Anticipating is also crucially important during these years. As you set boundaries for your adolescent, think ahead a few years. If you let your freshman son stay out until 1:00 a.m., how late will he want to stay out as a senior? If you let seventh graders have a coed party with few chaperones—after all, they're only twelve—how are you going to dial it back when they're sixteen? If you tell your daughter that she looks really cute in a skimpy tube top when she's in fifth grade, how can you then tell her it's too revealing when she's sixteen?

In a few years, your kids will be out on their own, making their own decisions about every aspect of their lives. Anticipate this by making sure they have lots of practice making decisions before they leave home. If they've never chosen their own breakfast or done their homework without prompting, how will they know how to take care of themselves? You've established boundaries to keep them safe; now, within those boundaries, give them the freedom to make their own choices and learn from their mistakes as well as their successes.

Teenagers' emotional brain centers are fully functional, while their prefrontal circuits are still "a work in process." In other words, the accelerator works great but the brake system isn't reliable. Treat your teen like an adult—after all, they're trying to be self-sufficient and make life-guiding decisions— but understand that at times they will act like children.

THE QUIET TIME PROGRAM

What's the very best advice a neuroscientist can give to the parents of teenagers? If you want to make sure they develop into intelligent, compassionate, successful, happy adults, encourage them to practice Transcendental Meditation. Our experience is that TM is a stress buster, an awareness builder, and a creativity booster. It's so effective that a number of schools have adopted it as part of their curriculum—calling it Quiet Time. James Dierke, executive vice president of the American Federation of School Administrators, said:

> *The Quiet Time program is the most powerful, effective program I've come across in my forty years as a public school educator. It is nourishing these children and providing them with an immensely valuable tool for life. It is saving lives.*

Quiet Time provides students with two fifteen-minute periods of Transcendental Meditation each day, to help balance their lives and improve their readiness to learn. It reduces stress, reduces alcohol and drug use, and dramatically improves academic performance, student wellness, and the school environment. Research shows that the Quiet Time program leads to higher graduation rates, better scores on standardized tests, and decreased burnout in teachers and administrators.

One of the main organizations responsible for the introduction of this program is the David Lynch Foundation, which has supported Quiet Time programs in private, charter, and public schools in the United States. For example, three schools in the San Francisco school district now offer the TM technique as part of their curriculum. One of them moved from the bottom in performance on standardized tests and the highest incidence of fights, expulsions, and student absences in the school district to one of the highest performances in the district. In two years, suspensions decreased by 86 percent; psychological distress (stress, anxiety, depression) decreased by 40 percent; and violent conflict decreased by 65 percent.

Transcendental Meditation can also help students diagnosed with attention deficit/hyperactivity disorder (ADHD). Dr. Travis conducted a six-month random assignment study to assess the effects of TM on students ages ten to fourteen years with ADHD. After the students practiced TM for six months, their parents reported significant improvements in their ability to focus on schoolwork, organizational abilities, ability to work independently, happiness, and quality of sleep. Their EEG patterns also changed. Children with ADHD have higher than normal activity in theta EEG (4–7 Hz) and lower activity in beta (15–30 Hz); doctors use this unique EEG pattern to help diagnose ADHD. After six months' TM practice, these students' EEG patterns were in the normal range. Note that TM did not mask symptoms or just help the children cope with ADHD, but actually normalized their brain functioning.

In Iowa, the Maharishi School (kindergarten through twelfth grade) has offered Consciousness-Based Education since 1975. This educational approach integrates Transcendental Meditation into the school day and teaches all the traditional subjects, including a college prep program in the upper school.

Every lesson is connected to the fundamental principles of the subject being taught, which in turn are related to the students' growing experience of consciousness within themselves. As a result, the students are bursting with creativity and energy—earning top recognition in everything from tennis to science fairs, from theater to National Merit Scholarships. Because all the students, teachers, and staff are practicing TM, the stress level at Maharishi School is very low, which provides an ideal environment for students to grow.

(Visit www.davidlynchfoundation.org to see the wide range of the application of the TM practice to address practical problems and www.maharishischooliowa.org to learn about the Maharishi School.)

CHAPTER 11

DHARMA PARENTING TOOLS:
The Young Adult Years,
Eighteen to Twenty-Five

IS EIGHTEEN SOMEHOW A MAGICAL age? Up to this point, you've taken care of everything for your children—food, clothing, a roof over their heads, the best possible schooling, vacations, *everything*. Suddenly, at around eighteen they go away to college or move out and find a job: *they're on their own*. Your son's or daughter's brain isn't very much different than it was a month ago, but now your soon-to-be-adult child has comparatively unlimited *freedom*. And without family structure to gently nudge them in the right directions, it's incredibly easy for them to go off track.

YOUR YOUNG ADULT'S BRAIN

From age eighteen through twenty-five, the brain finally completes its maturation. Neural pruning has established efficient pathways that will remain quite stable for the next decade, and as these pathways become more efficient, your young adult is feeling more settled and even. At the same time, neural connections throughout the brain have fully myelinated. Of course, pathways are created and myelination continues with each new life experience, but the basic structures are set. This maturity of brain functioning enables your child to make the transition from a teenager, who responds passionately to the world without much perception of consequences, to a thoughtful and increasingly responsible young adult. This remarkable growth is one of the reasons why car insurance rates go down at age twenty-five.

Between ages eighteen and twenty-five, you can almost see the change in brain functioning. In college freshmen, the brain's reward system has the upper hand and immediate gratification drives behavior. In college seniors, myelin has been added to prefrontal connections so interactions with the frontal "supervisory" areas are faster, enabling the frontal system to control emotional extremes. At this age, young people think more deeply about situations and act less on impulse. Rather than considering only their immediate circumstances, they are now able to take into account such abstract concepts as consequences and moral considerations *before* they act. They're beginning to develop their own code of behavior rather than thoughtlessly following rules set down by parents or teachers.

THINKING AND LEARNING

As brain connections become fully established, young adults begin to simultaneously consider competing answers to problems. They get better at abstract thinking and are more creative in solving problems. They can plan ahead more comprehensively and stick to a plan (or a budget) to see it through.

Young adults have so many options: college, a job in a new city, taking a "gap year" to live abroad or volunteer, staying near home and joining the family business, or learning a trade. Whichever route they choose, their prefrontal "CEO" connections are enhanced by these new organizational challenges and learning new skills. As they repeatedly adjust to new viewpoints, plan ahead, and consider larger issues around them, they're exercising the prefrontal executive circuits that support symbolic thinking. This type of thinking prompts even greater myelin formation around the frontal brain circuits, which in turn increases processing speed. It's synergistic: brain circuits mature and young adults begin to function as adults; in turn, new responsibilities and pursuits further stimulate the maturation process of their brains.

As these executive circuits develop, perception expands and deepens. Your more mature son or daughter learns how to think critically, work in groups, reflect upon and learn from experience, manage conflict, foresee consequences, and plan for the future. In short, young adults can begin to understand themselves and how they fit into the world around them.

APPLYING DHARMA PARENTING TOOLS DURING THE YOUNG ADULT YEARS

TOOL 1: DISCOVER YOUR OWN AND YOUR CHILD'S BRAIN/BODY TYPE

If you've been using the Dharma Parenting tools for a while, your almost fully grown child can probably assess and balance his own brain/body type. They may know how to read their pulse, and how to adjust their diet, behavior, and lifestyle accordingly. Now it's time for them to take responsibility for both their balanced and imbalanced brain and behavior. Of course, your parenting isn't quite finished yet—you'll still be called upon for occasional help—but what you mainly need to focus on is helping your children find their *own* creative solutions when problems arise.

If your young adult is a Vata brain/body type, being on his own in college or a new job will be a wonderland of possibilities. The Vata mind naturally springs from one fascinating new option to the next. His greatest challenge will be to identify priorities and actually *plan* how to accomplish everything that needs to be done—and then *stick to the plan*. This isn't so easy for Vata types, who can get caught up in creative endeavors—making music or a work of art, or decorating a new apartment or dorm room. They may tend to forget about less fascinating projects— that twenty-page history paper due tomorrow, or grocery shopping to fill the empty fridge. If they call you up, overwhelmed at the thought of everything they have to do, talk it through together in detail. Help them figure out what they absolutely need to get done (priorities), and the steps they need to take. They may need more than one pep talk from Mom or Dad to get through the crises. But take heart: if you keep coaching them, letting them do more and more of the planning each time, they'll eventually learn to organize their lives by themselves.

Pitta brain/body types are more than ready to take on the challenge of living away from home. Whether it's a new job, taking a gap year, or going to college, Pittas want to excel at everything. Their natural ability to focus will serve them well, but their competitive drive can make them overly assertive in the office or the classroom. Pitta types tend to be convinced that they know the right way to do just about everything, so they might jump in a little too quickly and too strongly, before they grasp the big picture. And if it happens that they don't excel—perhaps they received a B+ on a midterm, or their boss asked them to take it easy with the suggestions—they may feel crushed. If they call you with a tale of woe, remind them that they know what they need to do, and give them the chance to come up with the answer: stay in balance, get good rest, and eat the right food *on time* for their brain/body type. Appeal to their love of organization by suggesting that they set up a detailed schedule for themselves. If they live close enough, invite them home for a weekend to sleep in, away from the pressure of work or school.

Change is generally difficult for Kapha brain/body types, plus they tend to be dedicated homebodies, so they might not be as eager as Vatas and Pittas to set out on their own. Help them get used to the idea by starting early: months in advance bring up one issue they'll have to address—start with an easy one such as, "What new clothes do you think you'll need?" Then add the prospect of their new living situation, whether it's an apartment or having a roommate. If they're given time to adapt to the idea of a completely new situation, their strength and stability will usually serve them well in diverse and demanding circumstances. If they do go out of balance, however, their steadiness can be upset and they may become lethargic and withdrawn. If they call you feeling down in the dumps, remind them to keep stimulated and to get help from their friends.

"Daaaad! I love tutoring the kids, and I love the city, but my apartment mates are driving me nuts! Tammy spent forty-five minutes washing her hair when she knew that two other people needed to shower. And Janet spent hours decorating the living room yesterday

*and it looks great, but then she forgot about helping
to cook dinner and doing kitchen cleanup."*

*Alexis is taking a gap year before college, volunteer-
ing for AmeriCorps as an inner-city tutor. AmeriCorps
arranged for three volunteers to share an apartment,
but Alexis is worried that it's just not going to work
out. She's an only child and there's always been harmony at home, so she's never had to learn how to live
around people she's not 100 percent compatible with.*

Her father spends a minute or so sympathizing with her,
then brings up the concept of brain/body types. Since Alexis
understands that she's a Pitta type, he reminds her to try to
control her love of being in charge. Judging from Tammy's
and Janet's behavior, they decide that it's likely that Tammy is
a Kapha, while Janet is a Vata. Realizing this helps Alexis put
things in perspective. Not everyone is as focused as she is, but
each roommate has her own strengths to contribute, and the
three of them can work around each other's idiosyncrasies.
Tammy may be a little slow, but she can always be counted on
to do her part. Janet's creativity and liveliness add sparkle and
beauty to the group, and the others can gently remind her
about her responsibilities. Alexis will be able to keep them all
organized, as long as she doesn't try to be boss.

Young adults who are newly on their own are assaulted by
a barrage of decisions: exercise fiend or couch potato? party or
sleep? veggies or fast food? They have so many irons in the fire
that they can't balance all the demands made on them. One
way to keep all those irons hot is to build a bigger fire—increase their ability to handle challenges. This is the value of
transcending during meditation: to improve brain functioning and reduce stress.

The Value of Transcending

Transcending is a completely different type of experience—the experience of the inner Self, which is silent, vital, complete, and unbounded. Transcending occurs naturally during the practice of Transcendental Meditation and provides inner stability. From the brain's point of view, transcending increases both blood flow and alpha EEG coherence in those important prefrontal "CEO" areas where we do our decision making, planning, and creative problem solving.

Research at American University in Washington, DC, reported that three months of Transcendental Meditation decreases stress, anxiety, and depression; and increases brain integration, vitality, emotional and behavioral coping, creativity, and intelligence. Research at Maharishi University of Management (MUM), which has integrated the practice of the TM technique into its curriculum, reports increased practical intelligence, self-development, and happiness from freshman to senior years in its students, along with increases in brain integration. TM is great preparation for young adults who are going out on their own—to college or a new job.

NOTE FROM MOM

MAHARISHI UNIVERSITY OF MANAGEMENT

MUM's approach of Consciousness-Based Education is both innovative and unique.

Fully accredited to the doctoral level, the university offers an undergraduate liberal arts curriculum and specialized graduate programs. What makes MUM exceptional is its focus on the development of each student's inner and outer potential through the regular practice of the Transcendental Meditation program. The growth in creativity, awareness, and self-sufficiency produced by this technique is supported by extensive research, which shows distinct improvement in brain functioning and mental, physical, and emotional health.

Classes are taught on a one-month "block" system in which students take one full-time class each month. They don't have to manage the demands of several different subjects; instead, they go deeply into one subject at a time. Classes are small and professors work closely with the students.

The university is committed to a high quality of life and a sustainable global environment. MUM's consciousness-based approach to education attracts students who are aware of, and interested in, the development of consciousness—students whose goal is to be both successful and fulfilled in life. As one of the students said, "Everyone here seems to be wanting to improve themself, improve the world—or both." (For more information, see www.mum.edu.)

TOOL 2: HEAL YOURSELF

You've given 100 percent of yourself to your child. Now that they're grown, you can replenish your resources. Go back to beloved hobbies that may have fallen by the wayside. Read the book series that's been sitting on your shelf for so long. Participate in weekend and weeklong seminars and retreats to develop any and all parts of yourself. Rethink your daily routine and incorporate more deep rest, exercise, creativity, and time for yourself. Seek new challenges.

Mihaly Csikszentmihalyi, author of *Flow: The Psychology of Optimal Experience*, discusses the power of challenges to lead to optimal experience:

> *The best moments usually occur when a person's body or mind is stretched to its limits in a voluntary effort to accomplish something difficult and worthwhile. Optimal experience is thus something that we make happen. For a child, it could be placing with trembling fingers the last block on a tower she has built, higher than any she has built so far; for a swimmer, it could be trying to beat his own record; for a violinist, mastering an intricate musical passage. For each person there are thousands of opportunities, challenges to expand ourselves.*

We have mentioned that it's important to distinguish between *challenge* and *stress*. In a challenging situation, our brain stem secretes chemicals that speed up brain processing. We've all been challenged and we know how it feels: we're alert, creative ideas fill our mind, and we have lots of mental and physical energy. It's like riding a powerful wave—we can't wait for the next moment to come.

Under stress, the *opposite* occurs. The prefrontal executive circuits shut down, so we can no longer see the big picture or control our emotions. This is why we become emotional and make poor choices when we're under stress. And the long-term effect of stress is that it makes us more inhibited and less willing to engage in challenges. We begin to distrust others and interpret all situations as potentially threatening.

Strangely enough, a challenging activity yesterday can become overwhelming and stressful today. What's the difference? Lack of sleep reduces prefrontal blood flow so we have fewer resources to deal with the same situation—the challenge becomes overwhelming. This same process can happen if we indulge in alcohol or drugs. However, if we keep ourselves balanced and maintain good physical health, we can manage everyday stress. And we can go beyond merely coping with stress. Transcending can increase our creativity and vitality so that we can grow and flourish.

TOOL 3: ATTENTION AND APPRECIATION

Even though your older children are away from home, they'll still need your attention and appreciation. It's more important than ever to keep the lines of communication open, so stay in touch through e-mail, Skype, and the phone (you might go so far as to send a card or even write a letter). And remember that your young adult is never too old to receive a care package. Finally, be prepared—at any time of the day or night—for an urgent phone call. Your kids may not need your attention as often as when they were young, but when they need it, they need 100 percent.

Attention teaches values. Many children today are learning values and morals from the media, which loudly proclaims that alcohol is how you have fun and suggests that material wealth should be everyone's primary goal in life. To counteract this influence, you have to model the values you want your young adult to live. Also, speak with them about real issues—the environment, racial prejudice, social stratification, health care—all the things that you know are important for an adult to consider. Find out what's important to them and discuss those issues as well. Listen to their opinions, and let them have a chance to hear yours. But don't expect them to agree with you.

And remember that more than anyone else in the world, your kids know the difference between your words and your actions, so you'll want to be very straight and honest with them.

NOTE FROM MOM

E-CONNECTIONS

When your offspring begin to scatter all over the country—or the globe—take advantage of the Internet to keep in touch with everyone. Figure out a time when you can all connect once a week, either by group Skype or Google Chat—with video, of course, if your Internet is fast enough.

We chat on our laptops while we cook Sunday brunch in three different states. It's almost like cooking together at home.

Another good option for staying in touch is Facebook. We've created a secret group of only our immediate family members. We're always posting photos of excursions, recipes, requests for advice, and quite a few really bad puns. Probably our most common post is, "What time are we skyping Sunday?"

TOOL 4: ROUTINES

Routines have been a natural part of daily home life. Now, for the first time, your young adult has to figure out his own routines. Sometimes, especially in the beginning, it may seem hopeless to you—*will they ever figure out that they need more than five minutes between waking up and getting out the door?* There's not much you can do long distance except be sympathetic and offer an occasional lighthearted suggestion: "Well, if you don't want to get up before eight fifteen for your eight thirty class, you could always rig a zip line between your dorm room window and class." Be patient because they *will* figure it out in time: any natural inclination to be disorganized (the way they were in high school) is certain to be eventually corrected by their desire to do well on the job or in school.

TOOL 5: MELTDOWNS

Meltdowns *can* still happen. Young adults need the space to manage their own meltdowns, but it's good for you to be ready with a helping hand. If they're close enough, you might visit or they could come home for a weekend. The safety and comfort of a familiar and loving family environment will give them a chance to reflect more objectively on any problems they're facing. Your kids may be almost fully grown and have the final say, but you're still their life coach.

Dealing with the Stresses of Life

Sophie was a straight-A student in high school, and she got very excited when her first-choice college offered her a full academic scholarship. But when classes start in the fall, she discovers that she doesn't actually know how to study. School has always been so easy for her that she never had to develop good study habits. By the time she realizes that she's neither organized nor focused enough, half the semester is gone and she's way behind in all four classes. She's feeling a lot of stress, and panicking as her professors pile on more work.

Sophie is exhausted from staying up late studying and writing papers, and she seems to be getting further and further behind. She doesn't know which subject she should work on first: the history paper due in two days, the calculus exam at eight thirty on Monday morning, or the fifty pages of psych she's supposed to read for class tomorrow. Her scholarship has strict performance requirements; if she doesn't maintain a B average, it will be withdrawn, which would devastate her parents. For the past few weeks Sophie's had a recurring nightmare in which she slept through all her final exams. Every night she wakes up drenched in sweat and can't get back to sleep. Even more than she fears for her future, she dreads her parents finding out how badly she's let them down.

During their next Skype session, Sophie's parents, Rob and Elizabeth, notice that she looks tired and worried, with no energy or enthusiasm, and when they ask what's wrong, she finally tells them how poorly she's doing in her classes. This is a shock, but they've already realized that Sophie has not been her usual bright self for quite a while. Sophie asks if she can come home the following weekend to figure out her options in a familiar, less stressful setting.

Here's how Rob and Elizabeth use the six C's to deal with this young adult meltdown:

1. **Check in** with yourself

    This is Sophie's failure, not theirs. Naturally, they're concerned and disappointed, but they realize they need to carefully step back. This isn't about their disappointment; it's about getting Sophie back on track in college.

And Check in with Sophie.

Sophie's parents know their eighteen-year-old daughter well, and they have a good idea of how much advice and coaching she wants to hear from them. They carefully err on the side of noninterference by offering sympathy but not advice, until she asks for it.

2. **Comfort** your young adult

Rob and Elizabeth let Sophie know that they love her and support her, even though she feels that she's failed them. When she asks if she can come home for the weekend, they immediately agree. Sophie feels comforted knowing that she's no longer in this alone and can go to her parents for sympathy and advice if she needs it.

If your fledgling lives too far away for a trip home, you'll have to settle for giving them support via phone or video calls. Long distance makes it harder to judge how they're really feeling, but, again, if you're not sure how much to say, opt for less rather than more. And don't forget to send a care package: a surprise box of cookies or other treats always makes life seem a little more manageable.

3. **Change** your young adult's brain state

While she was still living at home, Sophie naturally turned to her parents for advice and support. In fact, most of the time she didn't even realize she was getting advice— it was just part of family discussion time over dinner. Now she needs to change to a more independent mode, looking ahead and planning how to meet all her new obligations.

Remember "scaffolding"? This is exactly what your newly fledged young adult needs: gradually reduce the intensity of your support so she can move from dependence to independence. From the ages of eighteen to twenty-five, as your young adult child's brain matures, is the time to consciously give less and less support and advice. You want to help just enough so the challenges don't become overwhelming and create stress. It may take some effort to hold back, but if you respect your child's growing autonomy, you'll have the satisfaction and delight of watching that child develop into a capable, thoughtful adult.

That's the big picture. Short term, Sophie needs to change her brain state from being stressed and indecisive to being rested and alert, clear thinking, and capable. This isn't going to happen if she's sitting in her room spinning her mental wheels. Her parents urge her to make an appointment to meet with her academic adviser right away; in fact, they wait on Skype while she sends the e-mail. The adviser, who has dealt with this problem many times before, will not be able to wave a magic wand and make it go away but can outline a number of options for Sophie to discuss with her parents when she is home the next weekend.

4. Choices

When Sophie was younger, giving her choices was an important step in dealing with a meltdown. Now that she's grown up somewhat and is away from home, choices are still a vital part of her processing, but Rob and Elizabeth realize that now she needs to come up with her own choices. If she wails, "What should I do?" they can simply ask, "What are your options?"

This is another opportunity for scaffolding. When your kids are first on their own, you can help them come up with possibilities, but be careful that you don't supply all the options—make them dig deep and see what creative solutions they can unearth. Then, *if they ask*, help them figure out which option is best. Suggest problem-solving strategies rather than specific solutions. Suggest that they make a list of pros and cons, discarding the option they like least until there's only one left. Urge them to take their time, if the situation allows, so they can fully consider all the possibilities and the consequences of their choices.

5. **Consequences**

Sophie's parents no longer enforce consequences for her; they realize that she now has to live with the consequences of her own decisions and actions, good or bad. In this case, Sophie hasn't been able to meet her academic requirements, and the consequences are clearly laid out. If Sophie starts trying to shift the blame onto her professors or the scholarship rules, her parents can gently nudge her toward a more constructive viewpoint: "Those are just the rules. It's up to you to avoid this situation in the future. If you need help, you can ask for it earlier." If Sophie learns the important life lesson that *she is accountable for her actions*, then failing one semester will have been a valuable and important step toward adulthood.

6. You are the **coach**

Your role as coach has changed. It's very tempting for Rob and Elizabeth to jump in and coach Sophie every step of the way, to make sure that she climbs out of the academic hole she's created. But they talk it over and decide that if they start micromanaging, it will be a signal to her that they don't think she can succeed on her own. When she comes home for the weekend, they help her consider her options and evolve a plan to get back on track academically, but they're very careful to offer suggestions *only* when she asks for them. At most they ask, "Will that work for you?" or "What will happen if you do that?" By the end of the weekend, they're both impressed and relieved with their daughter's maturity in handling this difficult situation, and confident that she'll work her way out of it.

TOOL 6: ANTICIPATE AND ADAPT

Scaffolding is the name of the game for the parents of young adults. You'll always be a parent, but you've almost finished most of your parenting job; the only thing left is to help your kids become independent instead of dependent. You want to constantly *anticipate* their next level of competence and independence by *decreasing* the amount of help and the number of suggestions you give them. As you gradually remove the scaffolding that's been in place for eighteen-plus years, they'll learn to take full responsibility for their lives.

What If They Move Back Home?

So . . . their first job doesn't quite work out and they need to come home for a while to regroup and find another position. Or they discover a tech job that would suit them perfectly but which requires a couple of years training at the local community college. Or they graduate from college and want to take a gap year before grad school, and living at home will allow them to save for a car and start repaying student loans.

Having your kids at home as young adults will give you an opportunity to *adapt* your style of parenting. At this point, they've been living as independent adults and have matured a great deal while living on their own. Do not allow them (*or yourself*) to revert to high school habits: depending on you for meals, laundry, and transportation. Sit down with them and set out guidelines so they're on adult terms with you: Do they pay rent? Meals? Gas? You will want to clearly stipulate how much they should help with chores and household expenses. They're too old for a curfew, but they should be careful not to disturb the family when they come in late. Don't treat them like children—treat them like responsible adults who contribute their fair share to the household.

You've helped your children grow in every area of life: physically, by keeping their body type balanced; mentally, by understanding and nurturing the development of their brain and mental abilities; and emotionally, with your constant attention and appreciation. You've encouraged them to unfold their own brilliance and inner creative potential. Now they step out on their own, confident, creative, and energetic, knowing they're unique in the world, and that by being true to themselves, true to their dharma, they can be happiest and contribute the most to society. Enjoy their successes, knowing that you have fulfilled your dharma as a parent.

APPENDICES

Maharishi Ayurveda Recommendations for Diet and Digestion

AYURVEDA IS DEFINED as the "science of life." It is the oldest system of natural medicine, with a profound knowledge of diagnosis and treatment of disease, as well as an extensive understanding of medicinal herbs and plants. Maharishi Ayurveda is Maharishi Mahesh Yogi's revival of this ancient system of natural medicine. It differs from Ayurveda in that it emphasizes the role of consciousness, which includes the technique of Transcendental Meditation, in all aspects of health. Maharishi gathered some of the greatest experts in Ayurveda and revived and transformed this extraordinary system of natural medicine so it could be taught and used by modern doctors.

In Maharishi Ayurveda, food is medicine. Maharishi Ayurveda has general recommendations for diet. In order to follow these recommendations, choose the diet of your dominant brain/body type.

MOST IDEAL FOODS FOR VATA TYPES

The general guideline is that sweet, sour, salty, heavy, oily, and hot foods are best for Vatas, while pungent, bitter, astringent, light, dry, and cold foods are not good.

1. **Best veggies:** asparagus, beets, cucumbers, green beans, okra, radishes, sweet potatoes, turnips, carrots, and artichokes. Other vegetables may be eaten in moderation if cooked in ghee (clarified butter) or extra-virgin olive oil. Avoid or reduce cabbage, sprouts, and raw vegetables.

2. **Best spices:** cardamom, cumin, ginger, cinnamon, salt, clove, basil, cilantro, fennel, nutmeg, oregano, sage, tarragon, thyme, a moderate amount of black pepper (also allspice, anise, asafetida, bay leaf, caraway, juniper berry, licorice root, mace, marjoram, mustard).

3. **Most organic dairy products** are highly recommended. Milk is easier for Vatas to digest when it is heated. The warmth also helps to balance their Vata.

4. **Favor rice, wheat, and oats** (cooked, not dry). And reduce consumption of corn (fresh corn on the cob in season, however, is great), millet, barley, buckwheat, and rye.

5. **Favor sweet, well-ripened fruits** such as apricots, plums, berries, melons, papayas, peaches, cherries, nectarines, and bananas. Also good are dates, figs, pineapples, mangoes, and avocados. If your child has digestive problems, fruits are best eaten lightly cooked, stewed, or sautéed.

6. Generally **all oils** are good.

7. **All natural sweeteners** are acceptable.

8. **Nuts and seeds** are fine, especially almonds.

9. Vata types are usually very sensitive to gas-producing foods such as beans. Bean such as chickpeas, mung beans, and tofu in small amounts are fine.

10. For nonvegetarians, favor fresh, organic chicken, turkey, fish, and eggs. Reduce or eliminate the consumption of red meat.

MOST IDEAL FOODS FOR PITTA TYPES

The general guideline is that sweet, bitter, astringent, cold, heavy, and dry foods are best for Pittas. However, pungent, sour, salty, and hot foods are not recommended.

1. **Best veggies:** asparagus, potatoes, sweet potatoes, leafy greens, broccoli, cauliflower, celery, okra, lettuce, green beans, peas, and zucchini. Also good are Brussels sprouts, cabbage, cucumbers, mushrooms, sprouts, and sweet peppers. Avoid or reduce tomatoes, hot peppers, onions, garlic, and hot radishes.

2. **All sweeteners** are okay in moderation, except for molasses and honey, which are heating to the system.

3. **Dairy** is helpful in balancing Pitta. Favor butter, ghee, milk, and ice cream. Since the sour taste can increase Pitta imbalance, sour or fermented products such as yogurt, sour cream, and cheese should be eaten sparingly.

4. **Organic grains such as wheat, rice, barley, and oats** are good. Reduce consumption of corn, rye, millet, and brown rice.

5. **Sweet and ripe fruits** like apples, grapes, melons, cherries, coconuts, avocados, mangoes, pineapples, figs, oranges, and plums are recommended. Also prunes, raisins, and figs are fine. Reduce or eliminate sour

fruits such as grapefruit, cranberries, lemons, and persimmons.

6. Pitta types need **seasonings that are soothing and cooling.** These include coriander, cilantro, cardamom, saffron, and fennel. Also turmeric, dill, and mint are fine. Spices such as ginger, black pepper, fenugreek, clove, salt, and mustard seed may be used sparingly. Completely *avoid* pungent hot spices such as chili peppers and cayenne.

7. Most nuts increase Pitta imbalance. Pumpkin seeds and sunflower seeds are all right.

8. **Favor coconut, olive, and sunflower oils.** Avoid or reduce almond, corn, safflower, and sesame oils.

9. **Favor mung beans and chickpeas.** Tofu and other soy products are all right in moderation, but the simpler and fresher the better.

10. For nonvegetarians, organic free-range chicken and turkey are preferable. Red meat and seafood increase Pitta imbalance and should be avoided.

MOST IDEAL FOODS FOR KAPHA TYPES

The general guideline is that pungent, bitter, astringent, light, hot, and dry foods are best for Kaphas. Sweet, sour, salty, heavy, oily, and cold foods are not recommended.

1. **All** vegetables are recommended, including asparagus, beets, broccoli, Brussels sprouts, cabbage, carrots, cauliflower, celery, eggplants, leafy greens, lettuce, mushrooms, okra, onions, peas, peppers, potatoes, spinach,

and sprouts. Reduce the consumption of such vegetables as sweet potatoes, tomatoes, cucumbers, and zucchini.

2. **Favor skim milk.** In general, reduce dairy intake, which tends to increase Kapha imbalance. You can, however, add small amounts of ghee, whole milk, and eggs to the menu.

3. **Honey** (raw, unheated, and organic) is the only sweetener that helps balance Kapha. Avoid all others.

4. **Favor grains such as barley, corn, millet, buckwheat, and rye.** Reduce intake of oats, rice, and wheat.

5. **Beans of all types** are good for Kaphas, except soybeans, fresh tofu products, and kidney beans.

6. **Fruits such as apples, apricots, cranberries, pears, and pomegranates** are good. Avoid or reduce fruits like avocados, bananas, pineapples, oranges, peaches, coconuts, melons, dates, figs, grapefruit, grapes, mangoes, papayas, plums, and pineapple.

7. **All spices except salt** are good for Kapha. Pungent spices like ginger, pepper, and mustard seed are good.

8. Except for pumpkin seeds and sunflower seeds, **reduce the intake** of all nuts and seeds.

9. Use **small** amounts of extra-virgin olive oil, ghee, almond oil, corn oil, sunflower oil, or safflower oil.

10. For nonvegetarians, favor fresh, organic free-range chicken and turkey. Limit or eliminate the consumption of red meat and seafood in general.

AYURVEDIC RECOMMENDATIONS FOR DIGESTION

Ayurveda has dietary recommendations but also gives recommendations to optimize digestion of our food.

1. Serve the main meal at noon when the digestive power of *agni* is the highest.

2. Make sure you have given enough time to digest one meal before starting the next. This avoids the production of *ama*, or undigested food, that is the source of disease in Ayurveda.

3. Start the meal with a digestive aid, which is made of ginger juice and lemon.

4. Avoid cold water, especially with ice, before, during, or after a meal, since it reduces the flames of digestion (*agni*). Instead, serve small amounts of room-temperature or warm water with the meal.

5. Always sit when eating and do not have other stimulation such as TV or phone conversations.

6. Conclude the meal with sitting for five minutes.

7. Do not eat honey that has been cooked. Only add honey to water that is not too hot. (You can test it by placing your pinky finger into the hot water and making sure you don't feel any pain.)

Self-Pulse

BECAUSE YOUR CARDIOVASCULAR system extends through-out your body—from your eyeballs to your liver to the joints of your big toe—it carries a wealth of information about how your physiology is functioning. Ayurvedic physicians are trained to "read" and decode this information by simply touching your wrist with three fingers. In this way they can assess balance and imbalance, and even detect disease.

You can learn a simplified method of self-pulse diagnosis to keep track of your state of balance/imbalance. And once you feel that you've mastered the technique, you can begin to read your children's pulse and help keep them in balance too. When they are old enough, they can also learn to take their own pulse.

Let's start with some definitions:

- **Wrist:** It's very important to note that women always feel the pulse that beats in their left wrist while men always feel the pulse in the right wrist. So in these instructions, *wrist* refers to a woman's left wrist or a man's right wrist.
- **Fingers:** A woman uses the fingertips of her right hand to feel her left wrist; a man uses the fingertips of

his left hand. So *fingers* and *hand* refer to a woman's right hand, or a man's left hand.

- **Styloid process:** This bony projection is about a finger's width below the base of your thumb—use your index finger to feel it sticking out. This is the reference point for figuring out where to place your fingers.

To take your pulse, extend your arm out in front of you—right arm for men, left for women—in a comfortable position, bent at the elbow, with your palm facing up. Now wrap your other hand around your wrist from behind. You are cradling the back of your wrist in the palm of your hand. Now curl the middle three fingers—index, middle, and ring fingers—over the top of your wrist.

Position your index finger below the prominent bony bump of the styloid process, so that it's just beside the edge of this bone.

Now line up your middle and ring fingers below your index finger so the three are touching each other easily side by side. And make sure the three fingers are completely level; raise your thumb and pinkie slightly so they're not touching your wrist. This is the position your fingers will always be in when you take your pulse.

Continue to slide your three fingers over and down your wrist about a quarter of an inch. Now you are ready to feel your pulse: very gently press all three fingers down until you can feel the pulse beating along the radial artery. It's important to use all three fingers together and make sure that your three fingertips are approximately level, sitting in a nice line at the same level of the pulse. When you can feel the beat of your pulse in any one or all of your fingertips, you will have reached the first stage of pulse reading.

Each of your three fingers corresponds to one of the three main brain/body types: the index finger for Vata; the middle finger for Pitta; the ring finger for Kapha. (Kapha may be so relaxed, or there may be so little Kapha, that it might be hard to feel it at all.)

Feel the pulse beneath each finger. (It can help to close your eyes.) Which finger feels the strongest pulse? Press down with all three fingers. Then as you slowly lift up, notice which finger receives the initial strongest impulse. For example, if you feel it strongest under your middle finger, that indicates that Pitta is strong.

You may or may not feel a pulsation beneath all three fingertips—this is perfectly normal. In fact, most people feel their pulse under one or two fingers; only a few feel it under all three. If you're predominately a Vata brain/body type, for example, the pulse under your index finger will be strong. You may feel little or nothing under the other two fingers. This doesn't necessarily mean that you're imbalanced—it does mean that at this time, your physiology has less Pitta fire or Kapha solidity in it.

What is the *quality* of your pulse? If it feels clear and the impulses seem coordinated—if it feels good to you overall—this indicates that your physiology is in good balance. If your pulse feels ragged or disconnected, with some impulses very weak while another is very pronounced, this tells you that you probably want to start getting yourself back in balance.

For example, if you feel Pitta pulsating very strongly under your index finger, it indicates that your Pitta is too strong and has invaded Vata's territory. It's time to stay cool and eat on time—but not at your favorite Mexican restaurant. If the pulse under your ring finger feels quick and irregular, you need to get your Vata in better balance. Slow down, stay out of the cold wind, and stick to a regular routine. If your Kapha feels very strong and dense under your middle finger, you may find that your digestion is sluggish and your mind is a bit dull. Balance that aggravated Kapha with some physical activity and fewer "heavy" foods such as desserts and mashed potatoes.

You can learn more about detecting balance and imbalance in your pulse by taking an online course at www.mum.edu/online.

Once you've mastered taking your own pulse, you can begin to take the pulse of your child. Please note that a mother uses the fingers of her left hand to take the pulse and a father uses his right. And take your daughter's pulse on her left wrist and your son's pulse on his right wrist. Don't worry that your fingers cover a large part of the child's arm—the process will still work. The gentle experience of taking your child's pulse will bring a soothing, balancing, and bonding influence between you, which can be very pleasant and nourishing for both parent and child.

Related Websites, Articles, and Books

Dharmaparenting.com
TM.org
Mum.edu
Davidlynchfoundation.org

Harung, H. S., and F. T. Travis. *Excellence Through Mind-Brain Development: The Secrets of World-Class Performers*. Gower, 2015.

Lynch, David. *Catching the Big Fish: Meditation, Consciousness, and Creativity*. Tarcher, 2007.

Rosenthal, Norman. *Transcendence: Healing and Transformation Through Transcendental Meditation*. Tarcher, 2011.

Roth, Robert. *Transcendental Meditation: Revised and Updated*. Primus, 1994.

Travis, Frederick. *The Brain Is a River, Not a Rock*. CreateSpace, 2012.

Travis, F. T., and R. K. Wallace. "Dosha Brain-Types: A Neural Model of Individual Differences." *Journal of Ayurveda and Integral Medicine* 6 (2015): 280–85.

Wallace, Robert Keith, PhD. *Maharishi Ayurveda and Vedic Technology: Creating Ideal Health for the Individual and World, Revised and Updated from The Physiology of Consciousness: Part 2*. Dharma Publications, 2016.

Wallace, Robert Keith, PhD. *The Neurophysiology of Enlightenment: How the Transcendental Meditation and TM-Sidhi Program Transform the Functioning of the Human Body, Updated and Revised.* Dharma Publications, 2016.

Wallace, Robert Keith, PhD. *Transcendental Meditation: A Scientist's Journey to Happiness, Health, and Peace, Adapted and Updated from The Physiology of Consciousness: Part I.* Dharma Publications, 2016.

Wallace, Robert Keith, PhD, and Lincoln Akin Norton. *An Introduction to Transcendental Meditation: Improve Your Brain Functioning, Create Ideal Health, and Gain Enlightenment Naturally, Easily, Effortlessly.* Dharma Publications, 2016.

Wallace, Samantha, with Robert Keith Wallace, PhD. *Dharma Health and Beauty: A User-Friendly Introduction to Ayurveda, Book One of the Smith Family Saga.* Dharma Publications, 2016.

Yogi, Maharishi Mahesh. *Science of Being and Art of Living: Transcendental Meditation.* Plume, 2001.

INDEX

Note: Page numbers in *italics* refer to charts.

after-school routines, 117–20
anger, 143, 148
anticipation and adaptation, 157–66
  about, 8
  and babies/toddlers, 189–91
  of changes in routines, 161–63
  of children's need for attention, 160–61
  of meltdowns, 163–65
  of need for self-care, 159–60
  and preteens/teens, 212, 233–34
  of responses of brain/body types, 157–59
  and school-age children, 210–12
  and young adult years, 253–54
appreciation
  about, 5
  anticipating need for, 160–61
  and babies/toddlers, 178–81
  and family meetings, 134
  and negative attention, 89
  and preteens/teens, 227–30
  and school-age children, 198–204
  and young adult years, 246–47
aromatherapy
  for parents, 50, 53, 62
  for sleep, 19, 72, 125
attachment relationship, 92–97
attention, 86–110
  about, 5
  anticipating need for, 160–61
  and attachment relationships, 92–97
  and babies/toddlers, 102–5, 178–81
  and coaching children, 154–55

and filtering information, 98
importance of, 92–93, 166
Maharishi's insights on, 98–99
and mirror neurons, 97–98
negative, 89, 108
power of, 89–90
and preteens/teens, 108, 227–30
quality of, 102
and school-age children, 105–7, 198–204
and values, 246–47
and young adult years, 246–47
attention deficit/hyperactivity disorder (ADHD), 235
authoritarian parenting, 214
authoritative parenting, 214

babies and toddlers (birth to three years), 169–93
  about, 9
  activities of, 175
  adapting to abilities of, 190
  altruism in, 95
  anticipating needs of, 189–90
  and attachment relationships, 93–94, 95
  and attention from parents, 102–5, 178–81
  brain development of, 169–70, 175, 178–81, *179*, 186, 191–93
  and childproofing, 190–91
  communication of, 95, 181–82
  holding, 192–93
  identifying brain/body types of, 174–75
  and meltdowns, 185–89
  and Pitta-Kapha combination, 48–49

strollers, 173–74
structured activities, 193, 200

Temper Thermometer, 148
terrible twos, 186–89
time-outs, 209
Transcendental Meditation (TM)
 anticipating opportunities for, 160
 benefits of, 12–13, 234–36, 243
 and children, 106, 120
 goals of, 80–81
 interruptions of, 177
 and Maharishi University of
  Management (MUM), 244
 of parents, 50, 64, 73–74, 80–81, 106
 and preteens/teens, 234–36
 as routine, 120
 and sleep, 73–74
 and value of transcending, 243

values, 246–47
Vata children, 20–24
 activities of, 175
 anticipating responses of, 158, 159
 and aromatherapy, 19
 and attention from parents, 104, 183
 as babies/toddlers, 174–75, 184–85
 and bedtime, 124
 characteristics of, 18
 development of, 179
 energy levels of, 22–23
 executive system of, 33
 and exercise, 115–16
 and family meetings, 136
 feelings of, 110
 and homework, 119
 identifying, 35, 174
 imbalances in, 23–24, 204
 and *Inside Out* characters, 91
 and Kapha children, 47–48
 and Kapha parents, 59
 and learning styles, 199
 mealtimes and diet of, 118, 183,
  257–59
 and meltdowns, 141, 144, 146, 164
 and Pitta children, 46–47
 and Pitta parents, 53–55
 at play, 43–44

 as preschoolers, 104
 as preteens/teens, 223, 226
 recommendations for, *39–40*
 and routines, 23, 113, 119, 124
 sensitivity of, 22
 and sleep, 184–85
 storybook-character example of, 37
 and Vata parents, 50–51
 as young adults, 240, 242
Vata parents, 49–52
 and exercise, 75
 and help with childcare, 69
 and school-age children, 105
 and sleep, 72
 and yoga, 76
vitamins and minerals, 83–84

walking, 74
wall chart for daily routines, 137–38
Winnie-the-Pooh storybook characters,
 37
work schedules, 102–3

yoga, 76–77
young adult years (eighteen to twenty-
 five years), 237–54
 about, 10
 anticipating developments in, 253–54
 and attention from parents, 246–47
 brain/body types of, 239–42
 and brain development, 237–38, 239
 with Kapha brain/body type, 46
 and meltdowns, 248–53
 with Pitta brain/body type, 45
 and Pitta-Kapha combination, 49
 and Pitta-Vata combinations, 47
 at play, 44, 45, 46
 and returning home, 253–54
 routines for, 247–48
 and scaffolding, 251, 253
 and self-care of parents, 244–46
 and stress, 248–53
 thinking and learning of, 238–39
 and value of transcending, 243
 with Vata brain/body type, 44
 and Vata-Kapha combination, 48

ABOUT THE AUTHORS

ROBERT KEITH WALLACE is a pioneering researcher on the physiology of consciousness. His research has inspired hundreds of studies on the benefits of meditation and other mind-body techniques. Dr. Wallace's findings have been published in *Science, American Journal of Physiology,* and *Scientific American.* He received his BS in physics and his PhD in physiology from UCLA and conducted postgraduate research at Harvard University. Dr. Wallace is founding president and member of the board of trustees of Maharishi University of Management (MUM) in Fairfield, Iowa. He is co-dean of the College of Perfect Health and professor and chairman of the Department of Physiology and Health.

FREDERICK TRAVIS is a world-renowned neuroscientist who has discovered brain wave patterns in children and young people that correlate with greater moral reasoning, happiness, emotional stability, and academic performance. His research has clarified brain patterns associated with the experience of higher states of consciousness. Dr. Travis has authored or co-authored seventy-five scientific papers, published in leading peer-reviewed journals. Dr. Travis received his Master of Science and PhD in psychology from Maharishi University of Management (MUM). After a two-year postdoctoral position at the University of California, Davis, he returned to MUM to direct the Center for Brain, Consciousness, and Cognition.